For dear Jo,
with gratitude for your support,
patience and excellent participation
in my classes!
love, Anish

The
FELDENKRAIS
METHOD®
Learning Through Movement

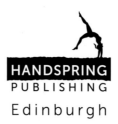

HANDSPRING
PUBLISHING

Edinburgh

The
FELDENKRAIS
METHOD®
Learning Through Movement

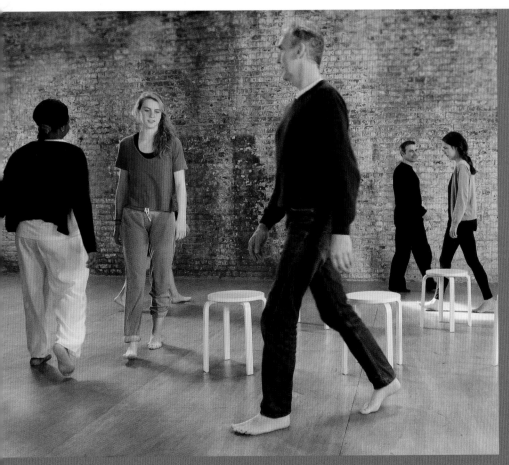

Contributors

Dorit Aharonov
Eilat Almagor
Ruthy Alon
Anat Baniel
Stacy Barrows
Deborah Bowes
Lisa Burrell
Karol Connors
Andrew Gibbons
Marina Gilman
Larry Goldfarb
Jeff Haller
Susan Hillier
Thomas Kampe
Paul Pui Wo Lee
Moti Nativ
Dwight Pargee
Lavinia Plonka
Donna Ray
Elinor Silverstein
Cliff Smyth
Linda Tellington-Jones
Matthew Zepelin

EDITORS STAFFAN ELGELID
CHRISH KRESGE

FOREWORD BY JERRY KARZEN

HANDSPRING PUBLISHING LIMITED
The Old Manse, Fountainhall,
Pencaitland, East Lothian
EH34 5EY, Scotland
Tel: +44 1875 341 859
Website: www.handspringpublishing.com

First published 2021 in the United Kingdom by Handspring Publishing

ISBN 978-1-912085-69-9
ISBN (Kindle eBook) 978-1-912085-70-5

British Library Cataloguing in Publication Data
A catalogue record for this book is available from the British Library
Library of Congress Cataloging in Publication Data
A catalog record for this book is available from the Library of Congress

Commissioning Editor Sarena Wolfaard
Project Manager Morven Dean
Designer Bruce Hogarth
Indexer Aptara, India
Typesetter Amnet, India
Printer Finidr, Czech Republic

The
Publisher's
policy is to use
paper manufactured
from sustainable forests

CONTENTS

CONTENTS *continued*

Part 3

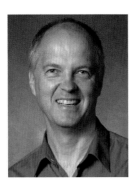

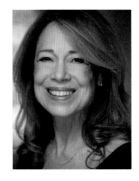

Dr Staffan Elgelid, PT, PhD, GCFP, C-IAYT, RYT-500, NBC-HWC

Staffan is a professor of physical therapy at Nazareth College in Rochester, NY. In addition to being a physical therapist, he is also a Certified Feldenkrais Practitioner and yoga therapist. Staffan teaches in yoga therapy programs, conducts workshops both nationally and internationally, and sees private clients.

When working with clients, Staffan's main focus is on using smart exercises, movements, and lifestyle changes to help build a robust and agile nervous system that allows them to learn new activities, enhance athletic performance, and withstand the stresses of daily life no matter what their age, level of activity, or situation.

Staffan is the co-author of *Yoga for Stress and Anxiety* and *Yoga for Active Adults*. He has also produced DVDs on topics such as core training and yoga for sports. He is on the Advisory Board of the IAYT and a board member of the Yoga Alliance.

Identification-differentiation-integration.com

Chrish Kresge, GCFP

Chrish is a Feldenkrais practitioner who works with people of all ages and backgrounds, using movement as the primary tool for improving function, coordination, awareness, self-image, voice, and overall health.

She has been teaching the Feldenkrais Method of somatic education for over 20 years in countries across the world, including the USA, Ghana, Morocco, France, and Nepal. In both her individual client work and group classes, Chrish aims to improve her students' lives by helping them learn to move in ways that are not only natural and easy but also enjoyable, using the brain's amazing neuroplastic capacity to reorganize the body. A former board member of the Feldenkrais Guild of North America, Chrish has chaired five national conferences.

Chrish maintains a private practice in Washington, DC and is also an actor, theater producer, and director.

Chrishkresge.com

Dorit Aharonov, PhD, GCFP
Dorit is a professor at the School of Computer Science and Engineering at the Hebrew University of Jerusalem, where her area of research is quantum computation. She has been practicing body-mind methods since 1994, including yoga and kung-fu, and is also a certified Feldenkrais practitioner. **cs.huji.ac.il/~doria**

Eilat Almagor, PhD, GCFT
Eilat is a Feldenkrais trainer and directs Feldenkrais professional trainings in Israel, Japan, and Italy. She uses Feldenkrais to work with children with special needs. Eilat has a degree in mathematics and physics, and a doctorate in neurophysiology. **restalittle.com/about-eilat**

Ruthy Alon, PhD (Hon), GCFT
Ruthy began studying with Moshe Feldenkrais in the 1950s and was one of thirteen students to attend his first training program (1968–1971) in Tel Aviv. She became a Feldenkrais trainer and directed professional trainings worldwide before creating her own Movement Intelligence program, comprising Bones for Life, Walk for Life, Chairs, Mindful Eating and Solutions. **movementintelligence.org**

Anat Baniel
Anat Baniel is founder of Anat Baniel Method® NeuroMovement® and author of *Move Into Life* and *Kids Beyond Limits*. NeuroMovement® evolved through Anat's unrelenting search for understanding her breakthrough outcomes with clients in terms of brain change. Anat provides private sessions, workshops, and practitioner training programs in the USA and internationally. **anatbanielmethod.com**

Stacy Barrows, DPT, GCFP, NCPT
Stacy is a doctor of physical therapy and certified both as a Feldenkrais practitioner and as a Pilates teacher. She is the inventor and author of the SMARTROLLER® self-care tools. Stacy owns SmartSomaticSolutions, a small integrative private practice in Southern California, and has taught internationally to health, wellness, and fitness professionals. **SmartSomaticSolutions.com**

Deborah Bowes, DPT, GCFT
Deborah is a Feldenkrais trainer and physical therapist based in San Francisco, CA who teaches in Feldenkrais training programs in the US and internationally. She is adjunct faculty at Saybrook University. Her doctoral research examined using *Awareness Through Movement* lessons to improve pelvic health. **FeldenkraisSF.com**

Lisa Burrell, DMA, GCFP
Lisa is a violinist, violist, public school string clinician, and certified Feldenkrais practitioner. She is on the faculty of Lone Star College in Houston, Texas. Her work focuses on implementing Feldenkrais-based pedagogy in music education to promote healthy playing and injury prevention and has been featured in the US, UK, France, Azerbaijan, and Portugal. **lisaburrellviolin.com**

Karol Connors, MPT, GCFP
Karol is a Feldenkrais practitioner and physiotherapist in Australia. She has over 20 years' experience in private practice and hospital rehabilitation, working with people who are living with neurological conditions and recovering from strokes. **baysidefeldenkrais.com.au**

Andrew Gibbons, MM, GCFP
Andrew is Feldenkrais practitioner with a practice in New York City and online. He teaches in professional training programs and works with high performers, world class musicians, and people who want to build their next body and brain. **bodyofknowledge.me**

Marina Gilman, MM, MA, CCC-SLP, GCFP
Marina has Masters' degrees in both voice and

communication disorders and is a Feldenkrais practitioner. She has incorporated the Feldenkrais Method into her work as a voice teacher in clinical practice at major medical centers, as well as in her published research on voice and the body. She is the author of *Body and Voice: Somatic Re-Education*.

Larry Goldfarb, PhD, GCFT
Movement scientist, multimedia author, cybernetician, and pioneering Feldenkrais teacher and trainer, Larry has been practicing Moshe's method for over 40 years, teaching it for nearly as long, and training others around the world for several decades. Larry is the founder and CEO of **mindinmotion-online.com**

Jeff Haller, PhD, GCFT
Jeff is a Feldenkrais trainer and regards the Feldenkrais Method as a pathway to the inner composure necessary for living a creative life in a challenging world. He studied directly with Dr Moshe Feldenkrais, graduating from the Amherst professional training course in 1983. Jeff trains Feldenkrais practitioners and sustains a private practice. **Insidemoves.org**

Susan Hillier, PhD, GCFP
Susan is a professor of neuroscience and rehabilitation at the University of South Australia, a Feldenkrais teacher, and also a Feldenkrais practitioner with a private practice in Adelaide. She is particularly inspired by working with people who have sustained movement challenges as a result of neurological injury. **people.unisa.edu.au/Susan.Hillier**

Thomas Kampe, PhD, GCFP
Thomas is a performing artist, researcher, and somatic educator. He is Professor of Somatic Performance and Education at Bath Spa University, UK, where he directs the Creative Corporealities Research Group. Thomas is

a Feldenkrais practitioner, a member of the Feldenkrais Guild UK, and guest editor of the *IFF Research Journal* Vol.6 (2019) Practices of Freedom: The Feldenkrais Method and Creativity. **bathspa.ac.uk**

Paul Pui Wo Lee, GCFP
Paul is a Feldenkrais practitioner, dancer, and rehearsal director who teaches in Europe and Hong Kong. He shares Feldenkrais with the ambition that people may continually uncover personal possibilities to possess the knowledge, and therefore dignity, to be healthily spectacular artists of their lives. **paulsfeldenkraisproject.com**

Moti Nativ, GCFP
Moti is a Feldenkrais practitioner and Master teacher of martial arts. He leads the Bujinkan Shiki (Awareness) dojo. Moti has researched the distinctive way that Moshe Feldenkrais became a judo expert. He teaches the Synergy of the Martial Arts and the Feldenkrais Method workshops all over the world and has served as president of the Israeli Feldenkrais Guild. **feldenkrais-ip.org**

Dwight Pargee, MSc, GCFP
As a lifelong athlete, martial artist, and coach with degrees in exercise physiology, sport science and biomechanics, Dwight finds great pleasure in working with high-performance athletes and those in the arts, refining high-level performance, dynamic balance, and neuromuscular learning. **facebook.com/Movaido**

Lavinia Plonka, GCFP, RSME
Lavinia is an assistant trainer for Feldenkrais practitioners and has been teaching in Asheville, NC as well as internationally for over 25 years. She is the author of several books, including *What Are You Afraid Of?* as well as audio programs on the Feldenkrais Method and its myriad applications. **laviniaplonka.com**

Donna Ray, MA, LMFT, GCFT
Donna is an internationally known teacher/trainer of the Feldenkrais Method, a psychotherapist and Interpersonal Neurobiology presenter. She imparts knowledge and experience from her 40 years of practice with tremendous vitality and insight. Donna's background in movement education, psychology, hypnotherapy, dance, and martial and expressive arts enables her to work in a variety of settings. DonnaRay.com

Tiffany Sankary, GCFP
Tiffany is an artist, Feldenkrais assistant trainer in Boston, and author of *Feldenkrais Illustrated: The Art of Learning*. She created an online comprehensive resource of hundreds of Feldenkrais lessons to do at home, curated from somatic teachers around the world, and other courses for physical, emotional, and creative growth. movementandcreativity.com

Elinor Silverstein, GCFP
Elinor is a Feldenkrais practitioner and holds degrees in biology and zoology. She has over 35 years' experience using the Feldenkrais Method and Tellington TTouch® to assist people with their healing process as they deal with serious nervous system disorders – both diagnosed and undiagnosed. onstickytopics.com

Cliff Smyth, PhD, NBC-HWC, GCFP
Cliff is a Feldenkrais practitioner at the Center for Movement and Awareness, San Francisco (www.feldenkraissf.com); faculty member in the Department of Mind-Body Medicine at Saybrook University; and teaches somatics at San Francisco State University. He is also a health and wellness coach, and editor of the *Feldenkrais Research Journal*. feldenkraisresearchjournal.org

Linda Tellington-Jones, PhD (Hon), GCFP
Linda's pioneering approach to working with animals, known as the Tellington Method, is taught in 37 countries. Her Tellington TTouch® for human healthcare has practitioners around the world. Linda has written 21 books on the Tellington Method and her work has been published in 16 languages. Ttouch.com/ttouchforyouonline.com/cellularwisdom

Matthew Zepelin, PhD
Matt Zepelin graduated from the Rocky Mountain 2 Feldenkrais training in 2014 and in 2018 completed a PhD dissertation on the history of somatics at the University of Colorado, Boulder. He still lives and practices in Boulder, working as an acquisitions editor for Shambhala Publications. Mattzepelin.com

(GCFP, Guild Certified Feldenkrais Practitioner; GCFT, Guild Certified Feldenkrais Trainer)

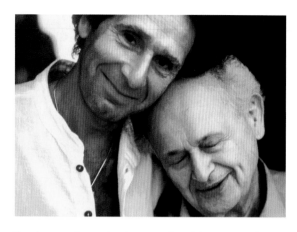

I've been given the honor of writing something about Moshe Feldenkrais and our relationship as an introduction to this book about the Feldenkrais Method and how it is used to augment and influence the generation of methods which have, in a way, grown out of it.

Moshe Feldenkrais was certainly, and in both senses of the word, the most curious person I have ever met. We would walk into a store for something and never get past the first few steps before his interest was piqued and he wandered off to examine everything that was near its entrance. The first time we sat down together to eat something, he started to eat off my plate without the usual formality of asking whether that would be OK – he just wanted to taste what I was eating. Moshe inspected every vehicle he got into; at a minimum this involved assessing how the windows and door worked, so if there was a crash he could easily get out. When visiting someone's home he might wander off into bedrooms or see where the back door was, simply because he was curious to see how these people lived.

Moshe was a survivor. His work about the human body, its musculoskeletal system, and its relationships centers around this aspect of his thinking. The coat he carried around with him had recording devices, extra batteries, all sorts of scissors, sewing materials, bandages, antibiotics, water purification tablets, and cash in numerous currencies, including Swiss and French francs and US dollars, in their thousands.

I think Moshe was the strong Jewish father figure I did not have. My biological father was a sweet, loving, very quiet Jewish man from the same region of the border between Russia and the Ukraine as Moshe. I sang Jewish songs to Moshe, which I had learned as a child. We held hands often, once for hours on a long car ride in Massachusetts… I was the son he never had. Anat Baniel once said that we carried on as a couple and should get married. One day in the training hall during the Amherst training, as he was looking for me (I was the program's organizer) he asked, "Where is my Jeddy Dahling?" The students made a t-shirt with that inscription on it for me.

We were two men doing a project about something we loved, and felt to be of importance, together. It was probably going to be his last training program, and I wanted desperately for it to succeed because of the importance I felt of what he had to offer to humanity. He never wanted to be audio-recorded because people would not know what he was thinking, feeling in his hands, or even seeing. So I was overjoyed when he finally agreed to my repeated requests to videotape the training and the many *Functional Integration* lessons he gave at the end of each training day.

There are, of course, many conversations and responses that I recall. Among these:

"How do you wish to be remembered for your work?" "*What will I care, I will be dead.*"

"If you had to do it over what would you like to have been or done?" *"An actor."*

Moshe's last definition of *Functional Integration* was: *"What a person needs; what the person will accept; what the person will use."*

I see this all the time in his lessons.

My friendship with him was a great privilege. What I miss most is his sweet, always courteous, always considerate love for me.

Jerry Karzen, GCFT is a Feldenkrais trainer who studied with Dr Moshe Feldenkrais in Tel Aviv from 1976 to 1983. During those years he was Feldenkrais' traveling companion, secretary, and close friend. Jerry organized and administered the last training program in Amherst and videotaped 95 percent of all existing tapes of private *Functional Integration* lessons Feldenkrais gave. Jerry has organized over 40 training programs in nine countries and is currently the educational director for Feldenkrais trainings in China, Germany, and Russia. **Jerrykarzen.com**

Pukalani, Hawaii, USA
March 2021

The Feldenkrais Method is the biggest basket available

I started out as a physical therapist, but soon felt confined by its limitations. I needed something that was more applicable to everything: individuals, groups, corporations, society... I needed something bigger. I tried other approaches, but always felt confined. Then, on a whim, I decided to enroll in a four-year professional Feldenkrais training program.

The Feldenkrais Method made me realize how we are defined and ruled by our habits. Habits that are ingrained as defaults in our nervous system. These habits are in the DNA of individuals, groups, corporations and whole cultures. They are sometimes formed over centuries in groups but can also develop rapidly in one person. Once habits are recognized, we can allow options and possibilities to emerge, but unless we first recognize them, we are just building patterns on patterns on patterns. Habits are different for everyone, and that is why a method with a big basket, such as the Feldenkrais Method, is needed.

This book is an example of how big the basket is. Contributors range from some of Moshe Feldenkrais' original students to more recent graduates. Even though I knew the basket was big, I was surprised to see how the practitioners who contributed to this book use the Feldenkrais Method in such unique and diverse ways. How the Feldenkrais Method can be used in schools, with athletes, and with animals are just some of the topics covered. I have learned so much from these practitioners who use the Feldenkrais Method on a daily basis to help individuals and groups enhance their potential and abilities.

Today I still root around in the basket and I always find something interesting to reflect about in the way we act in and interact with the world in similar and different ways. It never ceases to amaze me how big the basket is and how the Feldenkrais Method can accommodate for individuality, while at the same time allowing us to find our commonality. Enjoy this book and I hope it starts you rooting around and finding interesting things about yourself and the world around you.

Staffan Elgelid
Rochester, NY, USA
March 2021

How I discovered the Feldenkrais Method and why I stick with it

I encountered the Feldenkrais Method in 1988 while living in Cairo. My voice teacher, Raouf Zaidan, had taken some lessons with Carol Ann Clouston, another voice teacher based in the Egyptian capital, and he felt that Feldenkrais might help me overcome my habit of over-straining while singing. I made an appointment with Carol Ann who took me to a workshop taught by a visiting American Feldenkrais Practitioner, Eileen Bach Y Rita.

On the first day of the workshop we only did one lesson, mainly in standing, which turned out to be a variety of simple movements designed to explore how one turns around oneself. I recall being in the taxi on the way home afterwards, sobbing uncontrollably, relieved and excited about the possibility of learning to embody myself in new ways, and aware that I could release old postural and movement habits that no longer served me.

I continued voice lessons with Carol Ann, attended her weekly *Awareness Through Movement* classes, and also started individual *Functional Integration* lessons with her. I began to see dramatic changes, not only in the use of my voice but in the improved sense of myself and feelings of greater joy and agency over my life.

In the 1990s, I began the four-year Feldenkrais Professional training course run by Dr Frank Wildman in Boulder, Colorado, and, one year after graduating, I started my Feldenkrais practice in Rabat, Morocco, teaching *Awareness Through Movement* in English and French.

Five years later in Kathmandu, Nepal, I resumed my Feldenkrais practice and taught group classes above a charming bookstore. At the end of the classes, a young man working in the bookstore would appear with a tray of ginger tea for the students, unasked and unsolicited. The ginger tea after class became a long-standing tradition, which I uphold to this day with my students.

When my husband was diagnosed with aggressive melanoma, we returned to Washington, DC, where I settled after he passed away, established my Feldenkrais practice, and for 15 years have continued to be involved with the Method in many ways.

What makes me stay with Feldenkrais? I feel my capacity to respond healthily to the environment in which I live, regardless of its challenges, has become more robust; my ability to learn, improve and refine myself has increased; and I like myself more.

This work of improving the self-image, discovering internal strength and dignity, and the mental and physical flexibility that comes with it is something I would never give up. I am committed to sharing my learning with as many people as possible, and am deeply grateful each day to Moshe Feldenkrais and the extraordinary teachers with whom I have studied.

Chrish Kresge
Washington, DC, USA
March 2021

ACKNOWLEDGMENTS

First, I want to thank Sarena and everyone at Handspring Publishing for your support and friendship throughout the years. Thank you for your patience and for making this book possible.

Tied for first, I want to thank Chrish for being a great co-editor and having unbelievable patience during our Zoom calls. Without you and your hard work, this book would never have been born.

Third, too many to mention everyone, but…

To the chapter contributors, we owe you!

Matt and Jennifer Taylor: thanks for all your support, for the laughs and for always being there, and especially to Jennifer for putting up with me and Matt when I visit.

To Chris Bailey and family: You guys always bring me joy and are a constant reminder that the future is in good hands.

To Steve, Don, and everyone at Bloomsday: you're family. To Emma: Greatness awaits.

Tomas and Maria, my sisters in Sweden, and all my students, teachers, and friends: I love you all.

To my mentor YJ: Thanks for always taking time!

And of course, to Helena, who puts up with me every day. You bring me unspeakable joy and laughter. I can't thank you enough for being in my life.

Staffan Elgelid

I wish to acknowledge and thank each one of the 23 authors who contributed their time, creativity, and energy so generously and willingly toward the fruition of this book.

A huge thanks goes to Tiffany Sankary for the stunning images she contributed. Thank you also to the International *Feldenkrais*® Federation Archive for their permission to use photos from their rich and extensive archives.

Thank you to Lila Hurwitz, the editors' editor, as well as to Colin Davies for his helpful input. Great thanks must go to Doug Boltson for helping to write Ruthy Alon's chapter, to Ellen Soloway for her wise counsel and experience with all things Feldenkrais, and to Robert Burgess and Tracy Mulligan for their help with research. I'm grateful to Christian Buckard for supplying helpful personal details about Moshe Feldenkrais. I also wish to express my appreciation to the Feldenkrais Legacy Forum, John Tarr, Candy Conino, Chandler Stevens, Anastasi Siotas, Chris Murray, Mia Segal, and Larry Goldfarb for their contributions to the final chapter.

Thank you to my dear family and friends who patiently encouraged, advised, and listened; and to my coach Amy K. Musson, who helped guide me through the gestation of the book. Much gratitude and thanks to the superb Handspring Publishing team for their integrity and fine tuning; and of course to Staffan for being my co-author and friend. This has been an amazing experience.

Chrish Kresge

INTRODUCTION

This book is an overview of the Feldenkrais Method and the many ways that the method can be utilized in a variety of fields and settings. The topics of the book's chapters were originally chosen by us based on where we believed that the Feldenkrais Method had either made or could make an impact on the topic. We reached out to Feldenkrais practitioners and trainers with expertise in the selected fields, and we were overwhelmed by the response. Almost everyone we asked wanted to contribute to this book. Not only that, they also told us about other practitioners who were doing compelling work using the Feldenkrais Method. We followed up with several of the leads that we received and then sat down to decide how to proceed.

As we thought about the organization of the book, we realized that the first step was to divide it into three parts. The first would include chapters on the basic concepts behind the Feldenkrais Method: concepts that were important to Moshe Feldenkrais' development of the method. The second part would include examples of how the method is being used in specific settings, and the third would be about how the method can be used in learning and rehabilitation for people with specific conditions and difficulties.

We are well aware of the fact that many Feldenkrais practitioners do not feel that the method should be pigeonholed as being for specific conditions, but we nevertheless decided to shape the book based on that idea in order to make it easier to find a chapter that was relevant for the application that the reader was interested in. It was also a way to highlight with client cases the areas which some practitioners have chosen to specialize in. We hope that readers will find the way we

have organized the book to be a useful and easy way to find the information they are looking for.

We also felt it was a good choice to divide the book in this way based on the fact that the first part lays a very solid foundation for the rest of the book. Part 1 should be read carefully, and maybe repeatedly, as a way of understanding some of the foundational concepts of the Feldenkrais Method, such as learning through movement, the neurology of learning, and differentiation and integration. Once the reader has an appreciation of these, they will then be able to read the chapters in Parts 2 and 3 and understand how the authors applied those concepts to their specialized fields. If the book works in the way we envisage, the reader will also then be able to apply the concepts to both their own lives and those of their clients.

Something else that was important to us, and unique to this book, was to offer audio and video recordings of *Awareness Through Movement* lessons. Handspring Publishing made this possible by using QR codes that will take the reader to recordings of lessons that the author of the chapter teaches and that are relevant to their writings. So instead of having all of the instructions on the *Awareness Through Movement* lessons written in the book, audio and video lessons are included, enabling the reader to have an immediate kinesthetic experience of the topic of the chapter. This will not only deepen the understanding of the chapter but also give the reader a chance to develop and reflect on how their own habitual patterns influence their lives and shape their ideas.

It is the editors' and the contributors' hope that this book will bring more awareness of what the Feldenkrais Method is all about and how it can influence and enhance the lives of individuals and organizations. We are optimistic that, having read the book, more practitioners will be interested in writing about Feldenkrais, thereby raising the profile of somatic education in general and of the Feldenkrais Method in particular.

As we move through life at a blazing pace, with more information coming at us from all directions, it's important for us to be able to discern what is noise and what is relevant for our future. By engaging with the Feldenkrais Method, we can ensure that both individuals and organizations will act with integrity, discernment, and refinement, and build toward a sustainable future that includes the ideas that were important to Moshe Feldenkrais: concepts such as differentiation and integration, self-responsibility, life-long learning through movement, and maturity and the healthy development of individuals. As long as we keep learning and integrating our learning, whether as an individual or an organization, the future will continue to move toward solutions that lead to wholeness and transformation to benefit all of us. The choice is ours, dear reader, and it is our sincere hope that this book will be a first step towards a more integrated and resilient future for us all.

QR Codes of Audio and Video Files – Most of the chapters in this book have Audio mp3 or Video mp4 lessons accompanying them. You can access them by using the QR codes at the end of each chapter. Each clip has its own individual QR code.

The QR code can be scanned with a smartphone or tablet using an application for reading QR codes, freely available online. If you are using an iPad or iPhone, no additional application is required – simply open your camera and point it at the code (no need to take a picture). A notification should pop up, and by tapping it you will be taken to each audio or video file on the book's website, FeldenkraisMovementBook.com.

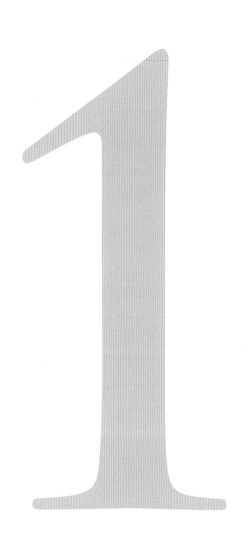

Moshe Pinchas Feldenkrais, educator and explorer of humankind, was born on May 6, 1904, in Slavuta, in the present-day Ukraine. He moved with his family to Baranovich (now in Belarus) in 1912, where he attended school, learned Hebrew, and received his Bar Mitzvah under the difficult battle conditions of World War I. At the end of the war, following the Balfour Declaration on the establishment of a Jewish state, Moshe, aged 14, left his family and embarked on a six-month journey to Palestine, arriving in December 1919. He knew already then that his education would be better served there.

Initially Feldenkrais worked as a laborer in the construction of Tel Aviv. At the age of 16, under the British Mandate in Palestine, Feldenkrais joined the Haganah, the Jewish self-defense organization, and after learning jiu-jitsu, devised his own self-defense method, which he taught to his fellow freedom fighters.

He soon enrolled at the Herzliya Hebrew Gymnasium (high school) in Tel Aviv, supporting himself by tutoring mathematics. After graduating from there in 1925, he worked as a cartographer for the British Mandatory Survey Office, making maps of Palestine, Egypt, and Syria.

Based on his experience and learning as a fighter and survivor, he later wrote and self-published a manual on self-defense, *Jiu-Jitsu and Self Defense* (1931). It was in 1929 that he badly injured his knee in a soccer match in Palestine, which also influenced his life's direction. He also read and translated into Hebrew *The Practice of Autosuggestion* by C.H. Brooks. This important work, to which he added two chapters, is about the power of conscious self-suggestion and self-hypnosis to improve any

condition, mental or physical.[1] He cared about his hard-working and fighting friends and understood that although their physical fitness was hugely important, their mental state was critical to their ability to survive.

Feldenkrais left Palestine and traveled to France in 1930, where he enrolled in the École Spéciale des Travaux Publics, a famous engineering school in Paris, graduating in 1933. Later he began working as a research assistant in the laboratories of Joliot-Curie at the Radium Institute in Paris while studying for his doctorate in engineering at the Sorbonne. The advent of World War II meant he did not receive his doctoral degree until the end of 1945.

His earlier interest in jiu-jitsu brought Feldenkrais into contact with the founder of judo, Jigoro Kano, whom he met in Paris in 1933. This seminal meeting led him to start judo training (Figure 1.1) and he went on to receive his black belt. Kano was impressed by Feldenkrais' skill and knowledge, and wanted him to be the conduit for introducing judo to France. Meeting Kano and judo embarked Feldenkrais on his life-long development of what became the Feldenkrais Method.

While in Paris in 1938, Feldenkrais married Yona Rubenstein, a renowned pediatrician, whom he got to know during his childhood and later in Tel Aviv when they both attended Herzliya Gymnasium. Yona had what was known as a congenital hip displacement (developmental dysplasia), and Feldenkrais used his skills and knowledge to help her regain better function (Reese 2015). Though they

---

1 Based on the French pharmacist and psychologist Émile Coué's original (1922) book, *Self-Mastery Through Conscious Autosuggestion* (Brooks 1922).

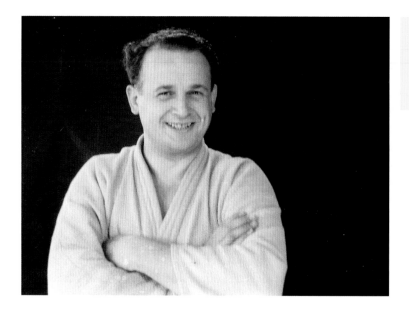

were married for only ten years, they remained life-long friends.

Escaping the Nazi advance on Paris in 1940, the couple fled to Britain, although not empty-handed. Feldenkrais carried with him heavy suitcases of secret documents connected to radiation research in Paris, which he took to the British Admiralty. Later on it was discovered that the documents contained, among other things, instructions on how to make phosphorus bombs. He was taken on as a scientific officer in the Admiralty, for whom he subsequently conducted anti-submarine research in Scotland from 1940 until the end of the war. He re-injured his knee both during the hurried escape from France and, later, while walking on submarine decks.

During this period, Feldenkrais taught judo and self-defense classes, which led him to publish *Judo: The Art of Defence and Attack*, and *Practical Unarmed Combat*.

Plagued again by his knee injury, however, and with no viable prospects for surgery, he became bedridden and began working in earnest to heal himself. By carefully observing the functioning of his knee and its relationship to the rest of his body through gentle movement and self-awareness, he began to develop a non-invasive system of movement and re-education that helped him overcome his injury. He wrote and gave lectures about his new ideas, began to teach experimental classes, and worked privately with colleagues. These lectures became the source of his next book, *Body and Mature Behavior*.

Feldenkrais remained in the UK after the war, moving to London in 1946, where he worked as a teacher and inventor, relying also on loans from friends. He took judo classes with Gunji Koizumi at the London Budokwai, sat on the international judo committee, and analyzed judo principles scientifically. He spent much time writing during these years (1947–48) and published his first full book on his method, *Body and Mature Behavior*, in 1949, and his final book on judo, *Higher Judo*, in 1952. During this period, he also studied and was influenced by the works of George Gurdjieff, F.M. Alexander, William Bates, and Heinrich Jacoby.

In February 1949 Moshe became a British citizen, but, nevertheless, he returned to Israel in September of the following year to direct the Israeli Army Department of Electronics. Around 1954 he moved permanently to Tel Aviv and, for the first time, made his living solely by teaching his method. He worked on the manuscript for *The Potent Self*, which he had begun in London in 1947, but which was not published until 1985, after his death. In this seminal work, Feldenkrais delves into the relationship between faulty posture, pain, and the underlying emotional mechanisms that lead to compulsive and dependent human behavior, and propounded his vision of how to achieve physical and mental wellness through the development of "authentic maturity."

Lest the reader think that Moshe was only interested in studying, learning, and developing his method, it seems important to add that he was also a very affable and fun-loving man. The life and soul of any gathering or party, he was curious about everything and everyone, loved the theater, and enjoyed good food.

Feldenkrais permanently located what he was now calling his *Awareness Through Movement* classes to a studio on Alexander Yanai Street in Tel Aviv. In 1956, he began giving lessons to Israeli Prime Minister, David Ben-Gurion, one result of which was that Ben-Gurion learned how to do a headstand, aged 71 (Figure 1.2).

Feldenkrais presented his work in Europe and the United States in the mid-1960s, publishing *Improving Ability: Theory and practice* (written originally in Hebrew and subsequently titled *Awareness through Movement: Health exercises for personal growth* in its 1972 English language edition). In 1968, a studio at 51 Nachmani Street in Tel Aviv became the permanent site for his private *Functional Integration* practice, and the location for his first teacher-training, which was given to a dozen students between 1969 and 1971.

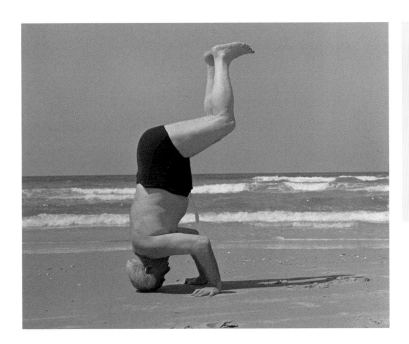

Figure 1.2
Prime Minister David Ben-Gurion of Israel performing a headstand on September 15th, 1957, aged 71, on Tel Aviv beach. He had many private lessons with Moshe Feldenkrais, and this was the first day he succeeded in standing on his head.

Courtesy of The Israel Museum, Jerusalem

After giving month-long training courses in his method internationally, Feldenkrais was invited to teach a large teacher-training program in San Francisco over four summers, starting in 1975. He also published *Body Awareness as Healing Therapy: The case of Nora* (1977), a fascinating study of his work with Nora, a woman who suffered a severe stroke, losing her ability to read and write.

It was a sign of how popular his method was becoming that in 1980 he began the 235-student Amherst teacher-training course in Amherst, Massachusetts. Unfortunately, however, Feldenkrais only taught the first two summers of the four-year program. After the second summer, while staying in Zurich with his close friends Lea and Michael Wolgensinger, he suffered a subdural hematoma. Dr Gazi Yasergil, a famous Turkish neurosurgeon and head of neurosurgery at the University of Zurich hospital, operated on him, suctioning out the old blood clot, probably acquired from his fighting days. At Feldenkrais' request, Anat Baniel flew to Switzerland to be with him and remained with him until he was well enough to return by

plane to Tel Aviv. He recovered and continued to work and teach from his home, but suffered several small strokes during this time. His book, *The Elusive Obvious,* was published in 1981, the year he stopped teaching publicly. Moshe Feldenkrais died in Tel Aviv on July 1, 1984.

Interview with Elinor

The following is an interview with Elinor Silverstein, a Guild Certified Feldenkrais Practitioner and Moshe Feldenkrais' cousin (Figure 1.3). Her mother, Hana Elter, spent some of her formative years living with Moshe's parents.

CHRISH: *Tell us about some of the memories that your mother, Hana Elter, shared with you about growing up with Moshe and his family.*

ELINOR: With the impending invasion of Russia and Poland by Nazi Germany, around 1932, my mother Hana, then five years old, was sent to live with her cousins, the Feldenkrais family, in Baranovich. Moshe's and Hana's mothers were cousins from his mother's side of the family (the Pshaters).

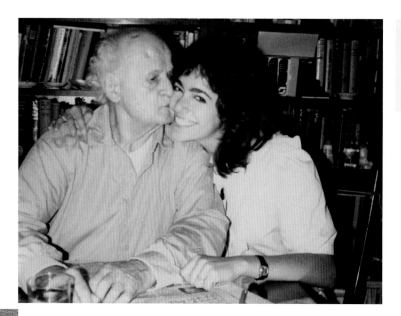

Figure 1.3
Moshe Feldenkrais and Elinor Silverstein, 1982.

Courtesy of Simon Elter

Hana lovingly referred to Aryeh Feldenkrais, Moshe's father, as Ari. He would invite her to sit with him and the local community of rabbis at the kitchen table on Shabbat to listen to stories from the Talmud about how we treat each other as human beings. He would say to her, "You are the future of the 'Land of Milk and Honey'... You will be the generation that makes the next generation." At that time, it was unusual for females to be invited to a table of men, particularly rabbis. However, Ari knew my mother was a precocious eight-year-old and that by bringing her to learn from her elders she would take this wisdom tradition to help others in need. She learned from Ari and the rabbis the importance of working together with the community for the greater good.

One day, Moshe's mother, Sheindel, was bathing little Hana. Hana saw tears flowing down her cheeks and asked why she was weeping. Sheindel responded, "Little Hanyetchka, my life isn't so easy. Here I am, a well-educated woman, and yet I must live at home and make my life for my husband. I am here to teach you, so that when you grow up you will have more choices than me, and your daughter will have more choices than you, and so forth. We will continue to raise our children to learn how to be free and live their lives to the fullest. You will remember this and learn. For now, we will always reach out to those who do not have and help them. So come, after your bath we will go and prepare soup for others."

Later on, in the Amherst Feldenkrais training in 1980, Moshe frequently talked about the turmoil of growing up, and the long-term issues that we carry with us into future relationships and situations. How many people love the idea of family and at the same time find it difficult to actually be with them? You have a deep desire to be loved by your family and be with them, and yet within 20 minutes of being back home, you understand why you just spent the last 10 years away. I would look around the expansive gymnasium where the training took place and see that this statement clearly resonated with a large majority of the other students.

Moshe's desire was to teach people how to be healthy, strong, independent human beings, capable of fully giving and receiving love. How do you raise a child that feels tended to, heard, and loved without dominating them? Instead, creating an environment that gives the child enough space to explore and always feel safe. Moshe gave many lessons to children during the Amherst training in 1980–81. There were those who could not leave their mom's arms, and those who were completely disconnected from everyone in the room. When he was working with a toddler, he would ask the mother to stay seated and not tend to her child's every need: he was setting up an environment for the child to feel safe and ready to learn. How could the toddler eventually crawl away from mom and know that she was not afraid or worried; rather that she was present and witnessing her child's process of learning in a safe environment? As he explained, "I want your child to find his own self-will. I want your child to have the freedom to crawl away from you and crawl back, knowing there is love and safety."

Moshe was committed to creating new generations of healthy people whose physical and emotional state was not dictated by past traumas such as those incurred from horrific wartime experiences. Generations who could live viable and full lives with the ability to have free choice in every moment.

Moshe's interpretation of health was the ability to be present in the world, enacting oneself with choice rather than reacting from a place of old personal habits. Health includes the ability to move freely in all five cardinal directions and back. He used this principle of reversibility by creating many *Awareness Through Movement* lessons highlighting this important concept.

Moshe also talked frequently about what it meant to respond rather than to react. He felt that getting over trauma was not just talking to someone about it, but that by feeling and becoming aware of our own body through movement, we could begin our own healing process. When we move with intention and the clarity of our self-image, we make positive changes in the brain, and when we make these changes, it allows us to respond meaningfully and thoughtfully instead of by being reactive.

I believe that the unity of mind and body is an objective reality. They are not just parts somehow related to each other, but an inseparable whole while functioning. A brain without a body could not think.

Feldenkrais 2010

You mentioned the strong influence that Moshe's mother, Sheindel, had on Moshe and his education, thinking, and evolution. Can you say more about that?

Education in the Pshater-Feldenkrais home was very important. Boys studied the Torah and the Talmud, and many became rabbis. After that basic education, they would also work to earn a living for their family. In the Feldenkrais family it was publishing; in the Pshater family it was the timber and luxury fabric business.

The Pshater women (Moshe's mother and aunt) were all intellectuals and well-educated. Their education was taken very seriously, as their parents held that without the knowledge of history and science, they would live lives of constant reiteration of the same story. Meaning, when we learn about history, we are less likely to repeat the mistakes that can lead to the annihilation of a culture. With clear knowledge of the past and present, we as a culture and human race are much less likely to repeat the history that created hatred, war, plague, and famine. This was the environment that Moshe Feldenkrais grew up in and is why, when he taught, he made sure to create an environment conducive to learning.

What is your earliest memory of Moshe? What was your relationship with Moshe like?

I was exposed to Moshe's teachings and philosophy throughout my childhood, even though I did not meet him until 1979. My mother was raised by Moshe's parents; however, it wasn't until the early 1950s that both of my parents began their studies with Moshe in Haifa, Israel. During the time he was teaching there, Moshe would come to their apartment every Friday evening to welcome in the Shabbat. The nights were filled with discussion and introspection about the challenging social and psychological conditions of people in a brand-new country after the war. They talked about how to bring healing to people after trauma and how to enhance their ability to create a new country that would allow future generations to grow and develop in a healthy and potent way.

My parents integrated what they learned from Moshe into their own lives, raising a family of physically and emotionally healthy children. From my mother, I learned the philosophy of his teaching; in particular, at a very young age my mother introduced me to Émile Coué's book, *Autosuggestion*, and how the technique of using my imagination and affirmations could help my joint and bone pain disappear. My mother had studied the work of Coué when she lived in Israel with my father.

From my father, Simon Elter, I received the beautiful hands-on work he learned from Moshe. My father had a gentle way of making my growing pains disappear so I could sleep at night.

My parents raised us with choice, being heard, witnessed, and learning to speak for ourselves. In an era when children were to be seen and not heard, we were raised with permission to disagree with our parents as long as it was done respectfully. In this way, when we grew up, we would never sit back and let things happen if we strongly disagreed with them. My father said, "As one individual, we might have a quiet voice, but when we all speak together and take action together, we can make changes in our lives and society."

My mother spoke with Moshe about my joining the San Francisco Feldenkrais teacher training in 1975, but I was only 16 at the time and it was the full-on hippie era – Moshe felt that there was no way he could protect me in an environment that had such free sexuality. It was the Haight-Ashbury era of "free love," and while Moshe had a reputation for being open about modern sexuality, he was, in fact, still quite old-fashioned.

Years later, during our Amherst training in 1980, when I was barely 20 years old, Moshe demonstrated his own "rules" about accepting behavior around free sexuality. No one was going to come between him and his family, as he told a suitor who had his hawk eye on me. Moshe walked toward him from across the room and said, "You know, she is my family, keep your distance." He looked deeply into this young man's eyes with a look that was undeniably protective of me. I responded that I could take good care of myself, but Moshe clearly knew better – this young Texan was in fact quite a ladies' man. I learned in this moment how family and love were

so dear to Moshe. My respect and admiration for him grew even more.

In our first year of the Amherst training, I went running up to Moshe during one of the breaks, excited beyond belief with the epiphany that every animal in zoos around the country deserved to be treated better than being confined to solitude on slabs of cement. All animals deserved to have freedom of movement and a life worth living. Moshe walked me out of the building onto a grassy field to introduce me to Linda Tellington-Jones (developer of Tellington TTouch® Training for animals) and said "Linda will be your new teacher from now and forever. You will always have each other." He was right. Linda became my teacher and friend, forever.

Moshe was kind, gentle, loving, and protective. I lived with him on Frug Street in Tel Aviv after his strokes, from 1981 to 1983, to continue my training directly with him. He was inquisitive, always asking how my day was and what lessons I had taught in my classes. When I was working with horses, he would greet me with enthusiasm, asking me how it went in the horse arena. What kind of horse did I work with? What did I do and how did the horse respond? With great enthusiasm I would say that the horse loved it. He would shake his head and then talk to me in detail about the difference between objective and subjective communication with people. We discussed at length the problem of anthropomorphizing our experiences with animals. He told me that once I was able to speak about my experience with animals objectively, then – and only then – would I be accepted by the scientific community. He told me how important this was, since I was both a biologist and a zoologist. I think if I had graduated from college with a degree in the humanities, he might have spoken to me differently.

What more can you say about how Moshe evolved his thinking and ideas?

I asked Moshe where he got so many of his diverse ideas. After all, he was not a neuroscientist, neurologist, or hypnotherapist. How did he know so much about subjects he was not trained in?

He said that every five years or so, a group of brilliant and like-minded people would gather at a local café in Tel Aviv or Paris and sip coffee and talk for a few days. Occasionally one person could not come but would recommend another. They would meet and discuss what each was doing. It was always based around how they could help and improve humanity, gently probing and picking each other's minds. They would go their separate ways with renewed curiosity and use these ideas to go even deeper into their own work. Then, about five years later they would meet again and compare notes about how they were helping to create more healthy, functioning societies. Moshe would smile, thinking of those days.

I will always be thankful to my dear cousin Moshe Feldenkrais for being a part of my life. And to his parents for taking part in raising my mother, who in turn helped my father through his post-traumatic stress after fighting many battles during and after World War II. My parents raised my brother and me to be true to ourselves and who we are as people, and to be happy and to know what that means. We had the privilege to grow up healthy in mind, body, and spirit, with the capacity to bring it to others. I am also thankful each and every day to have the honor of doing this very special work that encompasses who we are as truly magnificent human beings.

References

Feldenkrais, M. 1964. Mind and Body. *Systematics. The Journal of The Institute for the Comparative Study of History, Philosophy and the Sciences.* Available online: http://www.duversity.org/PDF/SYSMind%20and%20Body.pdf [Accessed November 2020].

Feldenkrais, M. 1981. *The Elusive Obvious.* Reprint, North Atlantic Books/Somatic Resources, San Francisco, CA, 2019.

Feldenkrais, M. 2010. Mind and Body. In: E. Beringer (ed.) *Embodied Wisdom: The collected papers of Moshe Feldenkrais*, pp. 27–44. North Atlantic Books, Berkeley, CA.

Reese, M. 2015. *Moshe Feldenkrais: A Life in Movement*, p. 147. ReeseKress Somatics Press, San Rafael, CA.

Other resources

Brooks, C.H. 1922. *The Practice of Autosuggestion by the Method of Emile Coué.* Dodd, Mead, New York. Project Gutenberg, EBook #29339, Release Date: July 7, 2009. https://www.gutenberg.org/files/29339/29339-h/29339-h.htm Download at: http://www.gutenberg.org/ebooks/29339

Vagal Nerve System *Awareness Through Movement* Video Lesson and Talk by Elinor Silverstein

My first exposure to Feldenkrais was in the early 1970s, and since that time it has not only been a source of endless fascination to me but, following my qualification as a Feldenkrais practitioner in 1983, also provided for me and my family.

Over the years, people have come to me to help them improve the quality of their life, recover from physical injury, emotional wounding, or issues that stop them from being more comfortable. I am a teacher at heart. What I provide for my students is the opportunity and environment to discover both their inherent ability to learn and the potential which, unknown to them, lies within them.

Inherent in every human being is the native ability to learn. What does it mean, to learn? According to Dr Moshe Feldenkrais, learning is the ability to acquire new behavior. When a child is born, she must learn how to navigate in the gravitational field she now inhabits: with the exception of primates, this is unlike other animal species, whose behavior is genetically patterned at birth.

Each child has a unique and individual path toward acquiring their ability to be in gravity – from organizing their eyes to see to making selective movements that appear at first to be random but eventually become a part of the way they negotiate rolling, turning, reaching, touching, bringing the world to them, and through their curiosity, moving into the world. During a short apprenticeship (usually 9–18 months) they move from lying to standing to toddling around and engaging in what they find interesting. Children accomplish these developmental movements not only in the field of gravity but in their "life field" – the home, family, culture, and society in which they will live. Each

child becomes conditioned by this life field, and that becomes their adaptation to life.

It does not take long before this environmental influence creates a sense of self, the self-image, with which a person identifies. As human beings, fragile in these early stages of environmental apprenticeship, they must depend on the support of those near them to provide for their personal needs for food, shelter, safety, and care. It is absolutely obvious that human children could not survive without being cared for; but they must develop and *internalize* the behavior that induces others to satisfy their needs. This is not a chapter on child development but a brief view into how people come to gain the behavior they adopt relative to the conditions into which they were born. A person cannot have any experiences other than personal ones; through learning they develop their own particular way of meeting the world.

A healthy nervous system will begin to make some behaviors invariant: in other words, develop habits. Habits are efficient, as they make it possible to live life with little forethought and without constant attention. Can you imagine how long it took you to hear sounds, learn to move your tongue in your mouth, touch your palate so you could replicate the sounds you heard and acquire the uniquely human ability to speak? Think how difficult it would be if you did not have the habit of speech, or of tying your shoelaces. What if you had to relearn these behaviors again and again? Most habits become deeply ingrained in our sense of ourselves. Our self-image operates with a preference in how we perceive, a preference in how we experience ourselves in movement, in how we relate to people and the environment, and in how we come to know ourselves.

But life is not perfect, and we adapt behavior in less than perfect circumstances. As we learn and are conditioned by the world, we suffer physical injuries, emotional wounds, and deficiencies in how we are supported or learn to be with ourselves. We acquire habits in everyday movements: how we sit, stand, breathe, look around. We come to rely on these deeply internalized habits of behavior to meet the world. In some cases, they work well, but in others our habits are cross-functional and weak. Habits occur as a necessity, being the quickest way to meet the moment before us. They become ingrained, and because every human being's need for self-preservation and safety is at a premium, habits are engaged before one is actually conscious of them arising. In a way, habits are reactions – not choices or responses – to the world we live in, and they take place compulsively. They are the only means we have to meet the moment. It is unfortunate, but many of us live our lives habitually, as we were conditioned by the world. Living life without being conscious of one's habits could be defined as neurosis. As Feldenkrais (1972, p. 3) said, "We act in accordance with our self-image… That self-image in turn governs the outcome of our every activity." If we have had a difficult journey in life, then we find ourselves anxious, insecure, or developing deeply habituated ways of acting to give us a sense of safety. It can be said that our neurosis, or inability to respond to life, is hidden in our muscular habit, and that our self-image is never equal to our real potential.

It is through this conditioning that the self-image people project comes to influence their sense of well-being: how they define success, the money they make, how they acquire the attention they need and the care they seek. Their self-confidence, joy, and happiness are tied to an external criterion found in their family values, culture, and society, and in what satisfies their internalized conditioned needs. People seek their sense of well-being from the world outside.

But if our habits of action are so regulated and compulsive that we are unable to consciously adapt our behavior to each new circumstance that befalls us, is it life? Our great capacity to learn has served to give us the means to survive in the world, but it is questionable if this way of just *surviving* in the world can be considered to be life. Feldenkrais said, "Life without movement is unthinkable" (Allen 2019). Of course, this is true from a biological point of view – we must move to survive – *but is living life through the lens of our conditioning realizing the human potential that rests within all of us?*

Make no mistake about it: without our conditioning and habit formation, we would not survive. Living in the world with a sense of purpose and meaning with which we can identify serves us. Deriving meaning for ourselves based on what we produce serves us and helps us maintain a sense of emotional safety.

When people come to my office for relief from pain from physical or emotional wounding, they are bearing the weight of the life they have confronted and lived in. They don't know that they really come to me to improve the quality of their life but often become increasingly aware of the underlying issues that affect their well-being. A person's injury is often an opportunity for growth, as it constrains them from being engaged in their habitual behavior long enough to question what they are doing with their life. I am happy when people come to realize this "elusive obvious," as Moshe Feldenkrais (2019) referred to it.

Not long ago I worked with a strong, athletic woman in her early 50s – let's call her Beverly – who

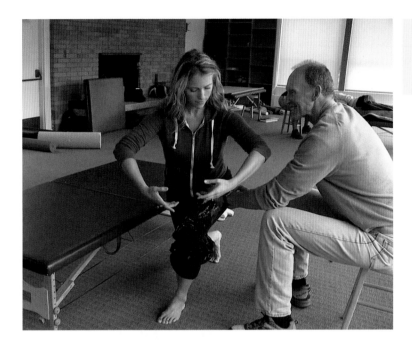

Figure 2.1
Jeff Haller working with a dancer.

Courtesy of Jeff Haller

had played soccer her entire adult life. She was experiencing severe knee pain because her lower leg was angled significantly outward and her foot was unable to support her knee when standing. She walked with a pronounced limp; each time she stood on her leg, her weight dropped into her knee. She could not find a clear path of support from the floor up through her skeleton. Each step carried a pain message with it – her internal means to protect herself. Pain was trying to help her stop damaging herself further until she could find a way to support herself safely.

We live in the field of gravity. Our nervous system seeks to remain upright and will do anything to stabilize us if we begin to fall. Orientation has primacy in our nervous system, along with self-preservation and procreation. As humans, we are designed to counteract gravity by organizing our movement intention to utilize our skeleton so force goes *up and through* our bones rather than shearing *across*

them. We all admire athletes, martial artists, and dancers who appear to float above the floor, who transfer the elastic forces from the ground up and through themselves easily.

Beverly was falling and shearing across her knee, which had been damaged through years of playing soccer. Pain, a product of the brain, was trying to protect her from further harm, but she was overriding the pain to play soccer. During our first lesson, I helped her learn how to organize herself so that her skeleton could support her more clearly. Afterward, she was able to walk around my office, and for most of the next week she walked without significant discomfort. In our second lesson (the sessions are called lessons because as Feldenkrais practitioners we create the environment for learning and acquiring new functional behavior), she was even more clearly capable of finding support through her leg. No pain was attached to the movement of walking.

Then what do you think she did, based on her prior conditioning? She had experienced two weeks of relief, so she decided to return to the soccer field and play an 80-minute game. Not surprisingly, she returned to my office in agony. I helped her regain her integrated sense of wholeness, support, and composure. When she sat up, her face was bright and open, the pain that had etched her face supplanted by calmness. She looked at me and said, "This is the happiest I have ever been in my life." Happiness and a sense of peace had been uncovered from within her.

And then she said, "But playing soccer is such a pleasure for me. I would hate to give it up." No doubt being embodied and playing with a team is a great experience and easy to identify with as a source of pleasure. It is easy to have these experiences become our self-worth, and this reward has been derived from an external source. We see, in this instant, two paradigms of living life before us. In one, we utilize outcomes driven by our will and conditioning as a basis of self-worth. In the other – the road less traveled, but deeply sought after and yearned for by many – is learning how to care for our most essential nature, to care for ourselves. For some, to give up the "pleasure" of their activities is too much. Others realize that their injury has been a part of their path into the inner domain and dimensions of self-realization and self-worth that are based on who they essentially are, not on what they can produce. This is the very nature of the midlife crisis for the self-made person, who after being successful looks back at their life and asks, "Is this all there is?"

In the course of my own development, I have asked this of myself many times. I was a former university athlete, a doctoral candidate in Transpersonal Psychology, and a black belt in aikido before I began training to become a Feldenkrais practitioner.

During this training with Dr Feldenkrais, I began to be conscious of how my self-worth was dependent on external successes.

Feldenkrais challenged me when he said to our class, "I take better care of you than you can take care of yourself." I thought, "How can this short round man take better care of me than I can?" It wasn't long after graduating from Feldenkrais' training that I opened a movement arts emporium in Seattle. The 9,000 square-foot space held classes in Feldenkrais *Awareness Through Movement*, yoga, tai chi, aikido, and old-school Japanese arts, in addition to the Feldenkrais Practitioner Training Program. Every week I would give 25–35 individual *Functional Integration* lessons, teach 7–10 Feldenkrais and aikido classes, teach workshops, and help administer the building. I was onsite for 16 hours a day. Slowly it dawned on me that I had no clue of how to take care of myself. I knew how to work hard with the purpose of bolstering my self-esteem. Sure, I was doing good work for people, but the real driving force for me was driven by my need for self-importance. It has taken years of ongoing and unending personal practice to keep discovering how to work from a place of love and care for myself as a basis for creating the *conditions* for learning with my current students.

What is learning and how do we create a context for it? When my students initially come for lessons, I ask them to imagine the future and project what would happen to them if they followed their current trajectory. If they keep doing what they're doing, what will their quality of life be like in five years' time, or in 25 years?

Everyone – especially those in pain who come to me as a last resort – can see their fate and the trajectory they are on. Unless they experience a new intervention that helps them with how they function in life, something that creates a new way for them to utilize their own natural inherent way of learning, they will be relegated to the predictable outcomes of their conditioned way of acting.

As a means to recover from our injuries, most of us participate in currently accepted modes of physical training and therapeutic exercises. These are for the most part prescriptive, repetitive directives that don't necessarily lead to changes in *behavior*. "Strength" is gained specific to the exercise practiced, but it does not lead to new patterns of motor planning and movement. If every person who did core strengthening exercises learned how to sit, stand, and walk more proficiently, they would be far more comfortable; however, the exercises they are doing do not lead to conscious changes in how they support themselves *in daily life activities*. Traditional exercises tend to lead to strengthening historic patterns of movement; the exercises are localized to strengthen and mobilize affected areas. But this works against the purpose of developing new refined ways of finding support for action and biological fitness.

Biological fitness is the unique capability of a person to meet change in an efficient way. A key ingredient of the Feldenkrais Method is that a student learns clear new patterns of action, movement, and support that are more efficient and effective for acting in gravity and in society.

I often ask my students this question: if they had only a half-hour to live, what would be the quality they would most like to experience? Other than the occasional few who would like to be doing their favorite adrenalin-filled activity, most people say they would like to be at peace, be tranquil, experience serenity, to be with their loved ones.

I wonder why these inherent human qualities are considered end-of-life qualities – why not live them now and for the rest of our lives? To me, living in tranquility is the essence of taking care of one's self.

It is the appreciation of who you are rather than what you can accomplish, and it is a very different quality of human freedom. We don't have to learn tranquility or peace: they are inherent qualities to be uncovered through learning to act as an individual unfettered by one's heritage, conditioning, and acquired compensations.

Living in tranquility or serenity does not mean living a life devoid of action and movement. Serenity can be expressed in the highest forms of human action. Observe the blissful look on an Olympic skier's face as they visualize the course they are about to run, the quiet they manifest in their preparations.

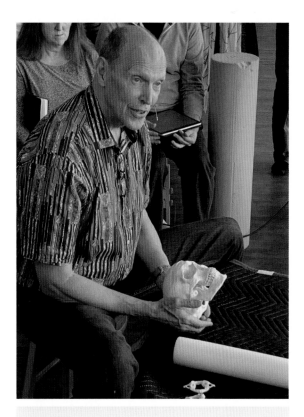

Figure 2.2
Jeff Haller demonstrating in a training program.

Courtesy of Jeff Haller

They seek to be efficient, not to work against themselves, and simply act with unadulterated intention.

In his book *Awareness Through Movement*, Feldenkrais (1972) spoke of three potential stages of learning for humankind. The first is the natural stage of learning; the second is the process of individuality; the third is method and profession. The first stage is the process by which people engage in the world and society. This is when they learn to eat, walk, take care of their daily needs, and be a part of a community.

Of those that acquire their means for daily survival through natural learning, only a few truly become individuals who define and develop unique talents and abilities. They evolve relative to the culture they are in but have a profound way of caring for something intrinsic within themselves from which their genius arises. They care for themselves and are internally driven to express their own creativity rather than hold fast to the strata of development that surround them.

The last stage, sadly, is the process by which individual creativity is then institutionalized and produced so that others can experience the advantages of one person's creativity – often to the detriment of true learning. Practices like aikido, yoga, tai chi, ballet, and modern dance all came from originators in their art, and their techniques were evolved so the work could be produced and experienced by many; but they can become rote practices at the expense of students developing their own individuality.

In a way, Moshe Feldenkrais came to us as an archetype of a person who can create the conditions for learning that invite people to reawaken their individual talents and uncover the potential that lies within. Feldenkrais was the rare person who comes along every few generations: he coalesced his Jewish heritage, academic studies, and judo training into a wisdom tradition, a process-oriented educational system that helps people recover their own individual abilities to care for themselves and unleash their own internal creativity.

A major neurophysiological theme that Feldenkrais was able to take advantage of is how our brain is an organ that utilizes *inhibition* in order to act. For example, our inner ear and vestibular system serve us by inhibiting unnecessary movements of the head, enabling our eyes to see accurately. Imagine how difficult it would be to see if you could not keep your head stable.

Consider the relationship between the older midbrain area, known as the limbic system, and the latest evolutionary development of the brain – the forebrain or prefrontal cortex. The limbic system is the internal system we rely on to provide us with a sense of safety in the world. We are obliged to monitor our sense of safety, especially if we have been emotionally wounded or physically harmed in the past. We tend to hang on to patterns of behavior that have served to protect us from harm and pain, and will continue to do so until something new is learned and we adopt more functional behaviors. Our prefrontal cortex interacts with the limbic system as each area of the brain serves to modulate the other. The propensities of the prefrontal cortex are:

- the ability to make distinctions and note differences (a necessary quality for learning)
- curiosity
- imagination
- spontaneity.

The limbic system will inhibit the brain from taking risks that are threatening to the known self-image. It can also keep the brain from learning new ways of doing and being in the world; often, if something new is learned it will be difficult to keep, as the familiar is more comfortable, even if it is ruining a person's life. On the other hand, the prefrontal cortex will inhibit and modulate the limbic system by engaging in new experiments that ask us to make distinctions and note differences. For example, if you wanted to learn wine tasting, which requires the ability to make fine distinctions in taste, you would need to be emotionally quiet so you could let the subtle tastes of the wine settle on your tongue. It would be impossible to make these distinctions – or to solve complex mathematical formulas – while emotionally agitated.

Feldenkrais understood the capacities of the prefrontal cortex to make the distinctions necessary for people to learn new behaviors, and recognized that therapeutic processes or exercises performed systematically and ritually don't necessarily lead to behavioral change.

A Feldenkrais practitioner helps people actualize their ability to learn by helping them turn their attention inward, so they can make concrete distinctions from which they become aware of how they habitually engage in movement. By asking questions and providing options, they guide the student into finding uncharted ways to act and move more efficiently with the minimal amount of muscular effort to achieve the greatest possible result. Our historic self-image is *hidden* within our muscular habit, but the student learns to remove unnecessary or parasitic habits of muscular action that interfere with a way of acting that is elegant and has physical integrity.

As you have read earlier, Feldenkrais developed two ways of working to help people learn. While to the outside observer they are two different activities, in essence they are both the same process – that of directing a person's attention so they make use

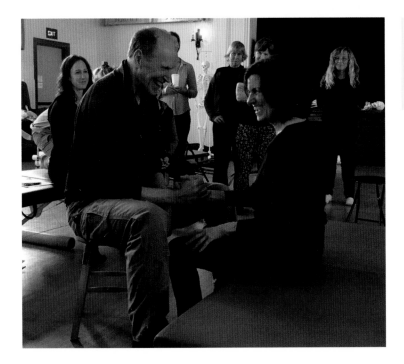

Figure 2.3
Jeff Haller teaching *Functional Integration.*

Courtesy of Jeff Haller

of the prefrontal cortex to uncover old patterns and create refinement in what they can do.

The woman who mistook an elevator for a carpet

A number of years ago I was teaching in Evanston, Illinois, giving *Functional Integration* lessons later in the day. My room was on the eighth floor of a hotel, and one evening I opened the door to find an absolute amazon of a woman with wild flaming-red hair wishing to attend my class. At over six feet tall and of athletic build, she nevertheless looked a bit tired from exercise. After introductions, I asked her why she looked frazzled and she replied that she had just climbed the stairs. When I asked her why, she told me, as incongruous as it seemed, that she was absolutely terrified of elevators.

Ostensibly, she had come to see me for a knee injury she had suffered playing volleyball. We worked together to discover how she could find clearer skeletal support through her knee and, after our lesson, she stood tall and self-possessed, with a truly regal bearing and a clear sense that her support through both legs had significantly improved.

As she was preparing to leave, I walked her toward the elevator door on the landing. She froze on the spot. Not only did her regal bearing dissolve but she began to fall in on herself, shrinking as if her proximity to the elevator diminished her. I asked her to back away from the elevator until she regained her sense of composure, and as she did this, her breath, height and fullness returned.

This gave me an insight, so I called the elevator back to the floor, held the door open, and asked her what she saw. Incredulous that I asked, she said, "I see an elevator." I answered that rather than an elevator, I saw a box. Buildings are essentially boxes with more boxes within, some of which happen to go up and down between floors. I asked her if she had ever been in a box like the one across from her before. She said, "No, I hate elevators." I asked her if she had ever been in a pantry, or a dressing room, or a toilet stall, or a closet, or a storage space, or even in a car, all of which are also boxes. As soon as her historic way of discriminating boxes was brought to her attention, she was able to change how she acted: she actually took steps forward, kept her integrity, and got into the elevator. Soon she even commandeered the controls, and we rode up and down before returning to my floor.

As we stood outside the elevator in parting, she had a profound look of realization and began sobbing. Through her tears she told me she had just realized that when she was four years old her brothers had rolled her up into a carpet and had left her there for a long period of time. She had associated her carpet experience with elevators ever since.

What was important to her was that her new state of composure made it possible for her to have a different way of meeting her fear reaction to elevators. Although it had been protecting her, it had also limited her freedom. When she could, of her own volition, go into and out of the elevator and command its ascent and descent, her need to protect herself dissolved... but not forever. I met her a few years later and she told me that she could still ride elevators, but to that day, she still had to pause a moment and make the conscious distinction to modulate her fear and remind herself that what was before her was an elevator, not a carpet. Without the contrasting sense of wholeness that she came to in our lesson, she would not have been able to walk into an elevator. She moved toward personal freedom, individuality, and a sense of her potential not bound by historic fear. And, oh yes, her knee was better too.

References

Allen, C. 2019. Body wisdom: Using Feldenkrais to Heal. *Alternative and Complementary Therapies* 25(1):9–11. Available online: http://doi.org/10.1089/act.2018.29198. cma

Feldenkrais, M. 1972. *Awareness Through Movement: Health exercises for personal growth.* Harper & Row, New York.

Feldenkrais, M. 2019. *The Elusive Obvious.* Reprint. North Atlantic Books/Somatic Resources, San Francisco, CA.

Other resources

Bernstein, N. 1996. Dexterity and its Development. In: M.L. Latash and M.T. Turvey (eds.) *Dexterity and Development.* L. Erlbaum Associates, Mahwah, NJ.

Doidge, N. 2007. *The Brain that Changes Itself: Stories of personal triumph from the frontiers of brain science.* Viking Books, New York.

Doidge, N. 2015. *The Brain's Way of Healing: Remarkable Discoveries and Recoveries from the Frontiers of Neuroplasticity.* Viking Books, New York.

Todd, M. 1980. *The Thinking Body.* Princeton Book Company, Trenton, NJ.

Rolling to Your Back While Flexing *Awareness Through Movement* Audio Lesson taught by Jeff Haller

The Importance of the Brain, Nervous System, and Body in Learning

3

Introduction

In order to be convinced that the brain, nervous system, and body are indeed important in learning, it is worthwhile spending some time understanding what these three terms mean. Several centuries ago, Descartes decided that the brain, as the seat of the mind, was distinct from the body. However, the brain is part of the body – indeed it is part of the nervous system – as much a part of the body as the lungs or the skeleton or the muscles. Rather than thinking about the separateness of these structures, it is more helpful to consider their interdependencies and how we use "all of us" to learn in an integrated way.

Definitions and anatomy

The nervous system refers to a series of structures that have the prime function of communication. The central nervous system (CNS) consists of the brain and the spinal cord. These two structures then divide into nerves (discrete paths or bundles of neural tissue), which connect them with every other organ of the body, and these nerves make up the peripheral nervous system (PNS). Figure 3.1 shows the key divisions in the nervous system.

The nerves that connect the brain/spinal cord and the muscles are known as *motor* nerves, whereas those connecting sensory receptors (in the skin, muscle, and so forth) to the brain are *sensory* nerves, and together these make up the so-called *voluntary* system.

A second division within the PNS is the autonomic nervous system (ANS), which has peripheral components operating in parallel to the voluntary system. The ANS used to be called the vegetative system, as it is largely responsible for unconscious or vegetative (visceral) functions, such as connecting the CNS with the smooth muscle of the viscera (abdominal organs), cardiac (heart) muscle, and glands throughout the body. It has two main branches – *sympathetic* and *parasympathetic* – which have been understood generally as fight/flight versus rest/digest functions. However, this is not entirely true, and perhaps a more accurate description of the two complementary (usually opposing or balancing) functions is that the sympathetic one enables the organism to respond and mobilize rapidly to situations, while the parasympathetic one offers a slower activation toward dampening functions, allowing repose and recovery.

Examples of functions that are either heightened (sympathetic) or dampened (parasympathetic) by the ANS include breathing, heart function, temperature regulation, digestion, urination, aspects of eye function, and activity in the reproductive organs. There are some functions that require both sympathetic and parasympathetic direction, such as aspects of sexual arousal and orgasm. A third division in the ANS has now been postulated – the enteric system – which is also involved in the functioning of the gut and lungs.

Interestingly, the ANS has both sensory and "motor" pathways like the voluntary system. This makes sense because, at the most simplistic level, you can consider the nervous system to connect structures that register information (sensory receptors) to the CNS for identification and analysis. These receptors are as diverse as sensing acid levels

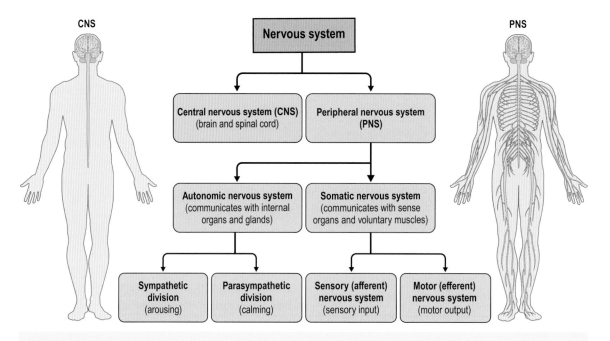

Figure 3.1
Divisions of the nervous system in humans.

Courtesy of Susan Hillier

in the gut or the pressure of touch on the skin, to detecting light in the retina of the eye or sound waves in the ears. The information they register is sent to the CNS as *afferent* (incoming) signals. In addition, the CNS connects to peripheral organs

that effect action, so it transmits *efferent* (outgoing) signals that activate end-organs – again these are diverse activities from regulating the beat of the heart, to secreting digestive enzymes in the gut, through to activating skeletal muscle for movement.

What is the relationship between sensing, thinking, acting, and feeling (that is to say, the emotions)? Consider how you experience an emotion. Think of the language you might use to describe it: hot under the collar, butterflies in your stomach, heart breaking. We experience feelings or emotions as a combination of thoughts or ideations, but also as sensations usually in the autonomically regulated organs. This is not surprising, because the key structures in the brain that are involved in emotional functions are the same as those regulating our organs.

Linking structures to functions

Why is it important to understand that the nervous system has this dual role of receiving information from internal and external environments and then transmitting messages for activity within the body? It is the most basic kind of learning: information is received, undergoes some kind of processing, then activity is enacted. And then the ongoing learning loop occurs: during and after the activity, the system senses its effect and reflects on whether it is beneficial. If the activity served a purpose, then potentially a memory of this loop will be encoded (sensory perception/information processing/activity) and learning has occurred. Whether this loop gets junked or survives depends on many factors (so-called neural Darwinism). Certainly, sleep is a major process that assists in either consolidating or deleting these daily "learning files."

Think about how you learn something. The process begins with one or more of your senses receiving information, which may be, for example, a visual image, verbal instructions, a temperature change, the sense of speeding through space, or a signature smell. Once the primary sense has been perceived and "made sense of" (you use memory to interpret the meaning and context, and maybe seek more information), you make a decision about a response. That response may be to commit the information to memory as knowledge or as a skill. Whether none or almost all of this process is conscious – some of it can be brought to consciousness – depends on the novelty and complexity of that information.

From this, it is clear that taking in information through one or more senses is the basis for learning. The body not only houses the sense-organs but directs or orients these organs so that they can more accurately detect (locate and interpret) the stimuli. Sense organs can detect signals that are either external to the body (exteroceptors) or internal (interoceptors). Without a moving body to maneuver the senses, we would be limited to receiving only those signals that come directly to us, and even then we would have trouble locating them precisely without the orientation actions that contrast the stimuli between two paired organs (two eyes, two ears, two nostrils, two hands).

Emerging research is strongly suggestive that multimodal (i.e., multiple) senses are more likely to induce learning. This is not to say that more is always better, as there is a suggestion that the senses must be congruent (all telling the same story) *and* relevant to the skill or knowledge being learned. This enhancement that occurs with multimodal sensing is based on associative mechanisms: the linking between the senses seems to produce richer engrams, or memories, of the skill or knowledge for better learning. However, we can make negative associations, such as the linking of pain "sensations" with the sense of certain movements, leading to kinesiophobia or fear of and reluctance to move. Learning is not always positive: emotions and feelings play a significant part in these associations and linkages.

> The structural architecture of the brain supports the importance of associations. Most senses have a known, dedicated region for primary processing, which is usually cortical; these somewhat modular areas, however, are neighbored and linked by even larger areas of *association cortices*. In the discipline of connectomics (the study of connectivity), breakthroughs in brain imaging are moving us away from making major assumptions about the size of specific brain regions in favor of measuring the strength of connection between them.

The physiological underpinnings of learning

What happens in the nervous system to support learning? This field has received a great deal of interest in recent decades and is known as neural plasticity or neuroplasticity. Neuro- or neural means part of the nervous system; plastic means change; and plasticity means changeability. There is still much to discover about the physiology of the brain's ability to change. What is clear is that this ability provides the underpinnings for learning; it has moved us out of the sphere of reflexive or hard-wired behaviors, turning us into a species that can adapt our behavior in response to a multitude of factors and can pass on individual learnings to other members of our species across time and space.

Learning, as described above, is contingent on a memory or series of associations being formed along the sensing–perceiving–cognition–action loop. Simplistically, these chains of associations are sited in the individual communication units of the nervous system, the neurons. These marvelous cells have a unique structure for their primary communication function – arm-like dendrites that receive incoming signals, a central processing body, and further arm-like branches or axons that transmit the signal to the next neuron (or end organ). Axons connect with the neighboring dendrites via special zones called synapses. These incredible little regions are stimulated by an electric current (action potential) traveling along the axon, and this message is interpreted in several ways and coded to produce the release of neurotransmitters that cross the synaptic gap and are picked up by the post-synaptic membrane on the dendrite of the next neuron. The types and amounts of neurotransmitter released and/or detected are significant in terms of the message being relayed (Figure 3.2).

Simplistically, neurotransmitters can either increase firing along neurons or prevent firing; that is to say, they can cause communication or they can shut it down. Being shut down (inhibited) is the more common state.

When learning occurs, the most likely thing is that there is a firing of a certain string of neurons via these synaptic connections, stimulating the production, release, and reception of neurotransmitters. Repeated firing (or practice) will most likely ensure that this neurotransmitter process will become more "permanent" (i.e., it becomes

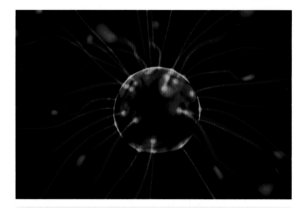

Figure 3.2
A representation of a neuron with associated dendrite and axon branches.

Photo by Josh Riemer on Unsplash

more likely that the same excitation/inhibition patterns will be reproduced again and again). Repetition matters because it leads to a state of *long-term potentiation*, which is thought to be the physiological underpinning of learning. (It is worth noting that the opposite– long term depression – can also occur, meaning a synaptic firing sequence is unlikely, i.e., is inhibited.)

Other ways that learning (plasticity) is thought to occur at the cellular or neuronal level is via an increase in the number of receptors, the awakening of unused synapses, or even the formation of new synapses.

It is not hard to imagine that strengthening these individual cellular linkages also occurs at a systems level, with larger groups of neurons starting to behave in concert and more likely to be involved in producing a particular thought or action. Therefore, interpreting complex sensory experiences becomes more likely and more refined with greater exposure. Neurons within a specific region are literally trained to be more specialized and nuanced in their function – and this process occurs along the learning loop. In the case of interpreting senses, there might be a greater specialization and differentiation in the auditory cortex for a musician who is learning to detect perfect pitch or in the olfactory cortex for a perfumier who can detect subtly different aromas. Further into the learning loop, a mnemonist (someone who can memorize extraordinary amounts of information) will use a vast quantity of associations – linking old connections with new to code a new sequence of information. Further on again into the action part of the loop, a fine artist may develop astonishing levels of differentiation in their motor (movement) cortex (and other areas of the motor system), which mean greater refinement in the activation and timing of finer levels of muscle units.

But what drives this reorganization at the level of major groups of neurons (called functional reorganization)? Researchers are still trying to find out predictors of this type of neuroplasticity. It is conjectured that the following factors are relevant:

- **amount and quality of practice** (as mentioned earlier and often linked to intensity and repetition), because of the use dependency of the neuronal firing patterns and the link to associativity;

- **level of meaning or relevance** that the skill or knowledge holds for the person trying to learn it (presumably something to do with motivation and level of association to other reward systems in the brain);

- **salience,** which means the degree to which something stands out or grabs the attention (and intention); and

- **specificity,** meaning that the training performed is what is learned; for example, practicing golf may not help your hockey game.

The phenomenon of learning

This brings us to the next important set of points. First let's re-cap: we know a bit about the brain and nervous system as important parts of the human body; we understand something of the way the brain/body learns by taking in sensory information, processing and encoding the knowledge or skills as memories for future thought and action; we know a little about the cellular basis for learning. But what is learning itself? Why do we learn? How does it manifest in our lives?

Learning has many definitions: the process for acquiring new skills and knowledge, the process for acquiring new behaviors, new ways of perceiving, new ways of thinking, and new ways of acting. There is also the addendum to the definition that there must be a relatively long-term duration to the change in skill or knowledge (it can't simply be a temporary thought or action), and that the cause of the change is from experience not from fatigue or drugs or other external manipulations.

Which brings us to the next point: what does learning mean to you? How do you know when you have learned something? Can you only tell if you have learned something if you pass the exam? The latter may only be a test of recall (memory) and therefore a rather crude way of determining whether you have learned something. Tests of comprehension, however, provide evidence that the knowledge you recall can be manipulated and discussed from different viewpoints (rather than regurgitating a strict word-for-word memory). What about the learning of activities? This can be demonstrated by reproducing the action with accuracy, like a dance, or with variations such as chess sequences. How else can we know if something has been learned other than an observable change in behavior? At this stage we cannot: it is inferred. There are experiments being conducted to demonstrate that brain connectivity or regions of interest change, but this is difficult to link accurately with the subtle changes that learning produces in skills and knowledge. So, we are left with our exams and tests, or, at an individual level, with noticing that something about the way we think or act is different to what it was before.

Over the years, research paradigms have explained different kinds of learning. Earlier types of learning were labeled associative as they had clear pairings or linkages. Consider the *classical conditioning* paradigm of linking a physiological stimulus (like the smell of dog food) with a non-meaningful stimulus (like the ringing of a bell). The first makes a dog salivate, then pairing the two together for a few repetitions links them and finally the ringing of the bell alone will cause the dog to salivate. We are now a bit more sophisticated – but not a lot! Much of our more subconscious learning happens this way.

Another associative learning model is the relatively simple linking of cause and effect. If we eat chocolate donuts, we feel happier. *Operant conditioning* then uses chocolate donuts as a reward to increase certain behaviors and withdrawing donuts, or replacing them with Brussels sprouts, can lead to decreasing behaviors (the reward and punishment learning cycle).

There is a postulated version of learning that is not associative – *habituation* and the opposite, *sensitization*. These processes happen at a neuronal level and can also be observed at a behavioral level. In some circumstances if a stimulus is repeated, it will cause the synaptic firing to lessen between neurons – they habituate or reduce communication. In other circumstances, a repeated stimulus will cause the synaptic connections to become sensitized or more likely to fire. The likelihood of the former or the latter happening is not well understood.

A further non-associative kind of learning is *perceptual learning* (sometimes called sensory learning). This is best understood as open-ended exploration, much as a child would do, simply gathering information with no intention of decision-making or taking action. Examples could include feeling, tasting, or poking objects for sheer discovery.

The final point to flesh out more is the role of *feedback* in the process of learning, which has been alluded to earlier. We take in stimuli (information), identify and process them, make decisions, and then we act. The process of acting involves our monitoring what is happening both during and after (knowledge of performance and knowledge of results, respectively). This is crucial for learning. It means we are continuously making sure that what we are doing is being improved and that next time we think that thought or do that action, it is more efficient. At least, theoretically. The feedback we monitor can either be intrinsic (i.e., comes from our own internal senses) or extrinsic (coming from external). Both are useful, but the main thing is that the feedback must be timely, accurate, and meaningful – and preferably repeatable. Using feedback to improve learning is fundamental so that the next time we plan an action we are *feeding forward* the best possible plan. How good we are at using feedback is one of the biggest factors in being an effective learner. The good news is that we can get better at all of it, at any age!

This was a quick tour around the brain, as part of the nervous system, which in turn is part of the body. All three are interacting in the context of an ever-changing environment and in the company of other embodied nervous systems (Figure 3.3). The importance of these interrelated systems in learning is hopefully now indisputable.

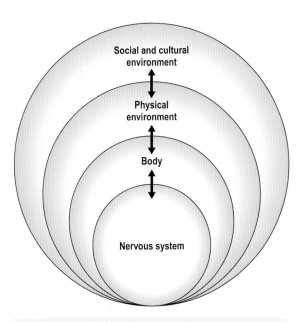

Figure 3.3
Learning is an interaction between the nervous system, via the body, with the environment.

Courtesy of Susan Hillier

Other resources

Mahadevan, V. 2018. Neuroanatomy: an overview. *Basic Science* 36(11):597–605.

Snell, R.S. 2018. *Clinical Neuroanatomy*, 9th edn. Lippincott, Williams and Wilkins, Philadelphia.

Introduction

To consider the training of Feldenkrais teachers is to contemplate the future of this neurophysical approach to learning. That's because the outlook for Moshe Feldenkrais' method will, in many ways, influence (if not determine) how well teacher training programs prepare trainees to successfully practice it.

In this chapter, we will explore what it means to practice the method successfully. We'll begin with the founder's approach, reviewing the ways in which Dr Feldenkrais trained others to teach his method before identifying the standard he set and the challenge this created for preparing future teachers. We'll take a look at what Feldenkrais teachers notice, understand, and do before considering how they learn these crucial sets of skills and the competencies that define the job.

The history of Feldenkrais training teachers

Every time Dr Feldenkrais trained others to teach his method, the number of participants in the program, the curriculum, and the aspects of the method he taught changed.

The first training process was a personal one: it started in the 1950s when Moshe took on Alexander teacher Mia Segal as an apprentice. They soon became co-investigators, ending up as close colleagues and collaborators. The second training, in Tel Aviv in the 1960s, consisted of 13 participants meeting with Moshe in the Feldenkrais Institute on Nachmani Street for a couple of hours a day, six days a week over the course of three years. The training focused exclusively on learning the hands-on aspect of the method; the trainees participated in Feldenkrais' weekly classes outside of the program.

The next training, which was only six weeks long and took place at the Esalen Institute in California in the early 1970s, focused primarily on what was then referred to as "the floor work." Moshe didn't do much more than demonstrate what was then referred to as "the table work," which meant giving the participants hands-on sessions followed by a talk on what he'd done. It was after conversations with the participants that Feldenkrais changed the terms for these two modalities from floor work and table work to *Awareness Through Movement* (ATM) classes and hands-on *Functional Integration* (FI) lessons, respectively.

Not satisfied with what he'd been able to impart to the participants in the next iteration of an ATM-oriented summer course (held in Berkeley, California), Feldenkrais then offered an extended multi-year program in San Francisco. Unlike Tel Aviv, Esalen, or Berkeley, this new program incorporated both modalities, interweaving long series of intertwined ATM lessons with demonstrations and practice sessions of hands-on skills. Unlike Tel Aviv – where there was a baker's dozen in attendance – the San Francisco group consisted of more than 70 participants. Also unlike Tel Aviv – where Moshe taught hands-on lessons as protocols, demonstrated the techniques to every trainee, and then they each practiced the technique on him – Feldenkrais switched from teaching by apprenticeship to training through demonstration and practice. He also made a transition from following an algorithmic approach to a more experiential and heuristic one, from following formulas to finding your way.

In 1983, Feldenkrais began a program that I was to join. There were over 200 participants at Hampshire College in Amherst, Massachusetts; the program consisted of nine-week summer sessions scheduled over four consecutive years (Figure 4.1). The ATM curriculum started with an exploration of the first movements of a newborn child, which were then followed by many more developmentally themed lessons. This was a stark contrast to San Francisco, where each summer's ATM series revolved around a different and distinct martial arts theme. The Amherst trainees were introduced to FI lessons by watching Feldenkrais working hands-on on video, receiving individual sessions from his faculty of assistants, observing a teacher from the San Francisco training (Mark Reese) work with Feldenkrais in class, and practicing ways of touching and noticing. When Feldenkrais became ill between the second and third summers, he appointed a faculty consisting of Mia Segal and a small group of graduates from the Tel Aviv and San Francisco programs to complete the final two years of instruction.

This ever-evolving approach to preparing others to teach his method demonstrates what is perhaps the defining aspect of Feldenkrais' approach:

he was continually refining his skill as an educator and continuously developing the method. Across decades of teaching lessons in classes, workshops, and teacher trainings, he returns to similar themes and compositions, yet he doesn't keep repeating the same limited vocabulary of movement. Instead, he explores how all kinds of activities – from early childhood development, everyday life, martial arts, the Chinese circus, yoga, children's games, other somatic approaches, and so on – can serve as laboratories for learning and become the source for an ever-expanding vocabulary, grammar, and syntax of meaningful action.

Notably, Moshe created and taught hundreds of different ATM lessons; he didn't teach the same lesson twice. Each lesson he taught and every training he conducted was a unique experiment: by delimiting specific variables, he defined a set of possibilities to explore, then made distinctions and divulged their connections. The way he taught was tailored to the place and the person or people he was teaching. Though he addressed individuals during classes only rarely, what he said and how he proceeded was directly in relation to the students in attendance.

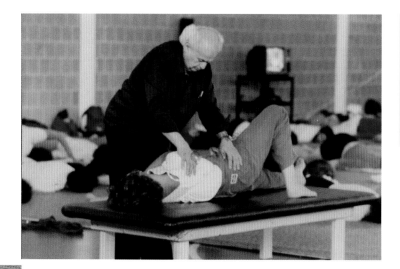

Figure 4.1
Moshe Feldenkrais teaching *Functional Integration* in Amherst, 1981.

Feldenkrais' trademark in-the-moment, interactive approach creates a conundrum for training teachers: if someone teaches exactly *what* Feldenkrais taught then they are not teaching *how* he taught. Certainly, there are classic lesson structures, foundational strategies, and established techniques that trainees need to learn, but these are the starting places, not the destination. While there's also plenty to learn from studying the transcripts and recordings of his lessons – and from doing those lessons as they were captured – to limit someone to doing this, and only this, is to condemn them to the role of an actor playing the part of the teacher (and to reduce the students to mere audience members, observers at a distance rather than implicated and engaged participants).

Repeating what's been done misses the dynamic aspect of Moshe's methodology. The aim of training programs is not to have graduates teach exactly what Feldenkrais taught; instead, we prepare them to educate in a fundamentally Feldenkraisian fashion.

Moshe's methodology

Whether we work with infants, toddlers, adolescents, adults, or seniors; no matter if people are dealing with pain, facing neurological impairment, wanting to prevent injuries, or looking to improve athletic or artistic performance, Feldenkrais teachers observe, comprehend, and respond in a common way. We'll start by defining *what* Feldenkrais teachers do and then examine *how* they learn the necessary skills, understanding, and abilities.

In the book he wrote to introduce his method, *Awareness Through Movement*, Feldenkrais (1972) declared that the method begins with action, distinguishing it from those that focus on emotion, thought, or sensation. He defined three aspects of the domain of action: timing, orientation, and manipulation. (This last term seems an odd choice to many; Feldenkrais, taking a systems perspective, was referring to how *the nervous system manipulates the skeleton through the action of the muscles*.) These three aspects provide a perspective to understanding intention-driven, perception-guided, self-organized orchestration of human motion – in a word, coordination – that defines the purview of the method.

A famously astute and insightful observer of action, Feldenkrais possessed a mime's uncanny ability to slip into someone's shadow, capturing the form and nuance of a person's kinetic "handwriting" perfectly. He was a veritable movement detective, someone who could unerringly uncover how people's ways of moving were the source of their troubles or challenges. Instead of tracing backward from a problem to its specific cause, he viewed local effects as the result of the global coordination of action. In this paradigm, problems are properties that emerge from patterns of action. This perspective is complementary to the way we usually think things happen. It involves, for instance, considering whether someone's back, neck, knee, or whatever might be hurting as a consequence of how they hold and move themselves, rather than automatically concluding that they must be moving this way because they're in pain.

We can trace this empirical approach to both Feldenkrais' professional life, first as a surveyor and then as an engineer, and his personal experience, studying jiu-jitsu and becoming a pioneer and proponent of judo in France. Back when Kipling's observation that East and West would never meet still held sway, Feldenkrais melded the ultimately European mechanical perspective of an engineer with an Asian martial arts master's embodied intelligence.

Instead of regarding movement as the sum of the actions of individual levers, Feldenkrais applied an engineer's insight to Jigoro Kano's brilliant revision of jiu-jitsu, modeling how the forces generated by muscles continuously orchestrate the overall moment-to-moment motion of the entire skeleton to create a biomechanical basis of his method. Even more importantly, the resulting model – which Feldenkrais utilized and taught but never fully explained – used judo's understanding of the human body's design for efficient and effective motion to define how we move when we move as well as we can.

By contrasting how someone is moving to their innate potential for ideal and efficient motion, we discover what is interfering with this person's potential for optimal coordination. This framework makes it possible for Feldenkrais teachers to accurately and reliably answer this crucial question: *How does the way someone moves and holds themself contribute to or cause the problem or challenge with which they want my assistance?*

It turns out that we rarely move as gracefully and well as we could. How we move isn't simply a matter of physical design, more a consequence of how our nervous system organizes, or coordinates, our action. From this neurophysical perspective, we observe that what we've already learned has become automatic, either through repeated intentional practice and training or as a result of the events that befall us and interfere with our potential. Asking this question reveals that our greatest limitations are not caused by what we can't do, but rather, by that which we can't stop doing.

Feldenkrais teachers see automatic – or habitual – movement as a sign of successful learning. Habits are a feature of your nervous system at work, not a failure of its design. We all rely on the autopilot and the habits it controls; they are necessarily central to being who you are and being able to do what you can do. The problem is not that we have habits – the

problem is that you, me, and the rest of us are not very good at updating the autopilot.

Why is that?

The outside of a habit, its motor aspect, is an action or behavior that repeats; the inside of a habit, what you notice – your sensory experience – is ruled by the perceptual process known as habituation, whereby constant stimuli disappear from awareness. *Consider this:* because you're familiar with how those nearest and dearest carry themselves, you can recognize friends or family members from far away. Yet you'd be hard-pressed to specify exactly what it is that makes it possible for others to identify you from a distance.

The consequence of habituation is that the things you do the most are the ones you're least likely to notice. This is a feature, not a failure: the advantage of not noticing what doesn't change is that you can be alert to what is changing, to news of difference. As difficult as it may be to appreciate at first, the fact is that habituation distorts your self-perception: your body image or, as Feldenkrais preferred, *self-image* – your very experience of your flesh and bones – like everyone else's, is more or less inaccurate, and you're unaware of this mismatch.

Consider the discrepancy between someone's subjective perception of their posture and their actual posture. Any attempt to correct how a student stands is experienced as something being "off," as an error signal that's soon corrected by the homeostatic readjustment that occurs almost immediately, unwittingly and unbeknownst to most everyone. The student's habit is as persistent as it is hidden by habituation.

Responding constructively to this mismatch between how we think we're moving and how we're actually moving demands the teacher's empathy, kindness, and diplomacy. Learning starts with *dishabituation*, that is, with discovering what's already there. After all, if you don't know what you're doing, how can you have any choice in the matter?

The job of Feldenkrais teachers is to coach their students in recognizing how they are already moving and acting as well as discovering new ways to coordinate their action. As the other chapters of this book reveal, we do this through two modalities: hands-on FI lessons and verbally guided ATM sessions, as workshops, group classes, or individual tutorials. While these two ways of working utilize different techniques, they share the same underlying tactics and strategies, the same emphasis on developing pragmatic abilities, and the same interpersonal, interactive pedagogical approach.

The contemporary curriculum

How do Feldenkrais teachers identify, cultivate, refine, integrate, and, eventually, master the distinct yet complementary sets of skills that make them effective movement detectives, neurophysical educators, and coordination coaches? Like the practice of the method, the training of teachers is, first and foremost, experiential.

From the beginning of their program trainees start learning how to benefit from ATM by developing their personal practice and making it relevant to their individual history and specific challenges. Then, after delving into the experience of the lessons, they begin to participate in an interactive, lively investigation into how and why ATM works. They do everything from simple introductory lessons to intricate series of interwoven ATMs (taken from Feldenkrais' training programs and public workshops that he taught). These add up to a total of some 400 ATMs over the course of the program.

To understand the body's design, trainees learn anatomy and biomechanics experientially: through their experience of doing ATM, by touching other students, and by "riding along" while someone else moves. They explore, learn, and refine a full range of hands-on techniques, delving into the how and when of each hands-on skill. Trainees also find out how to move themselves in ways that make each technique most effective and least likely to cause repetitive stress injuries. Where FI is concerned, in order to develop the ability to understand the techniques from the teacher's perspective, trainees coach each other in practicing hands-on skills and, eventually, giving FIs. Exchanging practice FI lessons under peer supervision provides the basis for giving lessons to the public under faculty supervision later.

Trainees take part in regular discussions with the entire class and, in some programs, in small groups (Figure 4.2). These discussions vary in style from question-and-answer periods to interactive dialogues and open-ended conversations on specific topics. They give participants a chance to grapple with difficult questions – those without providing pre-determined answers – and actively investigate them, learning how to deal with novel situations by employing Feldenkraisian reasoning.

Trainees participate in group exercises and learning labs designed to refine tactile, proprioceptive, and visual acuity, introduce key concepts, and foster cooperative learning. Working in small groups gives trainees the chance to learn *from* and *with* each other. They are crucial to developing the understanding and skills needed to teach FI and ATM. Participants are assigned activities such as observing a particular movement, practicing a specific technique, or analyzing a lesson. For example, in preparation to teach practice ATMs between class segments, they plan how to present their lessons and practice teaching sections to each other.

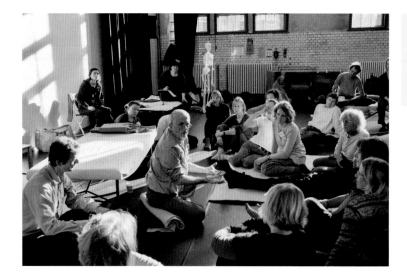

Figure 4.2
Larry Goldfarb in a class discussion.

Courtesy of Larry Goldfarb

Because *Awareness Through Movement* and *Functional Integration* rely on the same framework, trainees learn that they are two related aspects of the method, two sides of the same coin, each one illuminating the other. Didactic presentations and Socratic dialog supplement and deepen the experiential approach. The curriculum covers topics such as basic anatomy and kinesiology, pedagogy, systems theory, communication skills and other key concepts and approaches. Trainees learn about Feldenkrais' perspective and the history of the method by reading his written works, listening to and doing his ATM lessons, and watching videos of his FI sessions.

All along, trainees receive ongoing feedback to refine the touch that teaches. As part of the training, each receives a minimum of three individual FI lessons each year. On top of that, they see demonstration lessons given during class, watch lessons given to fellow trainees during non-class hours, and, in many training programs, can review the video recordings of class sessions between course meetings. To help trainees learn and track their progress, the educational director and faculty get to know each trainee. Observing the ways participants learn,

interact and practice in class, day by day, gives them the overview needed to assess the trainees' progress and nurture their development. That means that assessment, in the sense of watching and guiding, is an ongoing interactive aspect of the program, following an approach closer to vocational training instead of academic study.

Though there was no required standard curriculum during the first decades after Feldenkrais retired from training teachers, most programs followed the general outline and echoed the content of the early ones. More recently, training has retained the best aspects of the original programs while integrating advances in pedagogy, adult education, and contemporary technology, such as making recordings available online and offering opportunities for distance learning. For instance, in my teacher training programs we added a community-based ATM student-teaching project during the third year. Trainees prepare a class or, optimally, a series of classes, to present to an existing group or institution in their community. In this way, while still developing their skills, trainees have a teaching situation for testing their abilities, getting feedback,

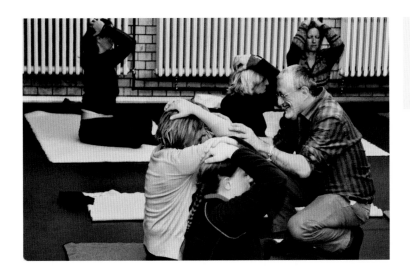

Figure 4.3
Larry Goldfarb teaching *Awareness Through Movement.*

Courtesy of Larry Goldfarb

and continuing to improve. They receive coaching from their study group and, during online office hours, from the educational director. The project gives them the opportunity to put what they've learned to work for the benefit of others, serves as a stepping-stone to being paid for teaching classes, and provides a beginning to becoming known as a Feldenkrais teacher.

Nowadays there are accredited Feldenkrais teacher training programs available all around the globe: in the Americas, Asia, Australia and New Zealand, Europe, the Middle East, and Russia. Building on the founder's original insight and continuing his tradition of innovation, these programs are preparing new generations of teachers to successfully help anyone interested in improving their resilience and coordination.

References

Feldenkrais, M. 1972. *Awareness Through Movement.* Harper & Row, New York.

Other resources

Checkland, P. 1999. *Systems Thinking, Systems Practice: Includes a 30-year retrospective.* Wiley, Hoboken, NJ.

Feldenkrais, M. 1993. *Body Awareness as Healing Therapy: The case of Nora,* 2nd edn. North Atlantic Books, Berkeley.

Hattie, J. 2008. *Visible Learning.* Routledge, Abingdon, UK.

Johnson, D.W., Johnson, R.T. 2018. *Cooperative Learning: The Foundation for Active Learning.* www.intechopen.com/books/active-learning-beyond-the-future/cooperative-learning-the-foundation-for-active-learning doi: 10.5772/intechopen.81086

Ryverant, Y. 2000. *Acquiring the Feldenkrais Profession.* El-Or, Tel Aviv.

Schön, D. 1984. *The Reflective Practitioner: How professionals think in action.* Basic Books, New York.

Von Foerster, H. 1981. *Observing Systems,* 2nd edn. Intersystems Publications, Seaside, CA.

A Comfortable Back *Awareness Through Movement* Audio Lesson taught by Larry Goldfarb

What is Integration? What is Differentiation? What did Feldenkrais mean by *Functional Integration*, one of the most important processes in his method? Why did Feldenkrais choose such difficult words to represent his work? As I continue to revisit Feldenkrais' terminology in my teaching and further study of the method, these words make me consider that complex problems often require more questions than answers, a process of thinking that Feldenkrais strived to ingrain in his students. In this chapter I will discuss Feldenkrais' use of the words function, differentiation, and integration in his lessons, lectures, writing, and discussions, reflecting the ways in which these have influenced my teaching and practice of the Feldenkrais Method.

Semiotics: the importance of words and symbols

Feldenkrais went to great lengths in his teaching and writing in order to avoid being misunderstood. He abhorred simplistic, reductionist thinking. He was almost obsessively devoted to talking "around" his main points in order to prevent his students from fixating on isolated examples. In the summer of 1975, for example, he made the point to his San Francisco training students early in their first year: "I said I would tell you everything. But I must do so in a roundabout way for all those people who are accustomed only to talking and therefore misled by language as if language were thinking." (Feldenkrais 1975–1977, June 19) In verbal explanation, as much as in the experiential practice of his work, Feldenkrais felt that the "successive approximation" of understanding of complex ideas was far more important than defining terminology or creating principles. He said that

principles and axioms were often broken as soon as they were stated.

In exploring multiple fields of study to find answers to his own questions, Feldenkrais developed a particular interest in semiotics – the use of symbolism and imagery in language across disciplines – often citing the semiotic work of Levi Strauss and Ferdinand Saussere (Feldenkrais and Pribram 1975). He used crossover language from mathematics, evolution, and phylogeny, neurophysiology, and cognitive studies and psychology in various contexts. Unsurprisingly, the terms function, differentiation, and integration have precise, but not identical, definitions in each of these areas of study. While Feldenkrais often referenced examples from each field to illustrate these terms, he strictly maintained that no single definition encompassed the totality of his thinking. Thus, using language that was common to all of these fields allowed him to express something broader than each field of thought could offer individually.

Semantics: the importance of intuition and felt sense

Feldenkrais believed in the importance of feeling and sensing long before the formation of an idea or thought, and even longer before a concept could be verbalized. Learning begins with experience. Felt sense, however, was not only important to Feldenkrais in terms of taking in sensory information in response to movement, but also in the semantic, visceral way that great discoveries are made. Einstein said of his Special Theory of Relativity:

A new idea comes suddenly and in a rather intuitive way. That means it is not reached by conscious logical conclusions. But, thinking it through afterwards, you can always discover the reasons which have led you unconsciously to your guess and you will find a logical way to justify it. Intuition is nothing but the outcome of earlier intellectual experience.

cited in Stachel 2001, p. 89

Likewise in mathematics, observation is sensed, seen, felt and heard first; a formula is derived, and the proof comes later, and often long after that its proof is reworked in search of greater elegance, clarity, or refinement.

Feldenkrais was particularly drawn to other thinkers who crossed the traditional boundaries of their own disciplines in order to make sense of complex ideas. These include, but are not limited to, Karl Pribram, neurobiology and psychology; Fritz Perls, Gestalt therapy; Milton Erikson, hypnosis; Margaret Mead, anthropology; and René Leriche, surgery, neurology, and medicine. They were among many like-minded influences who crossed over into other disciplines in search of ideas and language that could help them more clearly organize and communicate their own processes, allowing them to create new disciplines and modes of discovery.

As Feldenkrais began to evolve in communicating his ideas using terminology like function, differentiation, and integration to a larger audience, he often gravitated toward the ideas of these crossover thinkers to translate his semantic knowledge into something understandable and replicable. In addition to exploring the particular fields from which Feldenkrais' terminology is directly derived, this chapter will also look at the ways in which he borrowed ideas from "hybrid" thinkers in order to translate important semantic, or felt and experienced, ideas into language.

Mathematics

After pursuing his course of study in mathematics at the Herzliya Gymnasium, Feldenkrais won a competitive position in the Survey Office in Jaffa, drafting maps of Palestine for the British government. In Jaffa he immersed himself in his first practical applications of calculus, trigonometry, and Gaussian geometry (Reese 2015). In his teaching and work with clients, Feldenkrais drew many of his analogies for structure and function in learning from these forms of complex mathematics. He credited this early work experience as foundational in understanding human function through numerical models and mathematics, among his wide array of perspectives (Reese 2015).

In mathematics, a function is a relationship between inputs and outputs, with each input determining a specific output. The relationship between Fahrenheit and Celsius, for example, is a simple linear function. With linear functions we can determine the exact change in an output based on a change in an input: if you plug in a temperature in Fahrenheit to the function $C = (F - 32) \times \frac{5}{9}$ you get a corresponding temperature in Celsius. Many early and inaccurate models of learning and brain function were conceived using simple functions involving direct connections between input and output involving the sensorimotor cortex (Feldenkrais and Pribram 1975).

The mathematics of calculus, which employs the devices of differentiation and integration so central to Feldenkrais' work, evolved in order to study more complex, non-linear relationships. Calculus is often called the mathematics of the infinitesimal, because it involves a strategy of parsing smaller relationships in a process of "successive approximation" in order to understand more intricate relationships between inputs and outputs.

During Feldenkrais' tenure in the Survey Office, he worked with principles of infinitesimal approximation in helping calculate land mass for accurate real estate values (Reese 2015). His work involved converting highly varied three-dimensional terrain into two-dimensional map forms. He examined small segments of land for changes in elevation and compared these with spherically plotted coordinates of longitude and latitude in order to estimate, with increasing accuracy, the ratio of each plot of land to the whole of the region.

In calculus, *differentiation* involves examining increasingly smaller segments of a complex function in order to approximate the rate of change of the output with respect to a change in the input. Imagine Feldenkrais surveying bits of land over plots of 100 square miles, then 50, then 10, and so on, and comparing these to known coordinates.

The inverse of differentiation is known as *functional integration*. This is where the progressively smaller segmentation is reconstructed, or added together, and examined in the context of a larger segment of the function. Imagine how the estimate of the land values might be more accurately represented in the 100-square-mile area after examining the smaller segments in more detail.

In mathematics, complex functions are represented by infinite curves, which are then studied through parsing (differentiating) parts of that curve into smaller and smaller rectangles to approximate the area under that curve. As we can see in Figure 5.1, as the rectangles become smaller in width and are added together (integration), the approximation of the area under the curve grows successively closer to the actual area.

Feldenkrais often used the analogies of complex function in mathematics to illustrate how his method could be used to refine human function through learning (Feldenkrais and Pribram 1975). Like the varied and changing terrain of the territory Feldenkrais studied in cartography, he recognized not only the sophistication but also the ever-changing

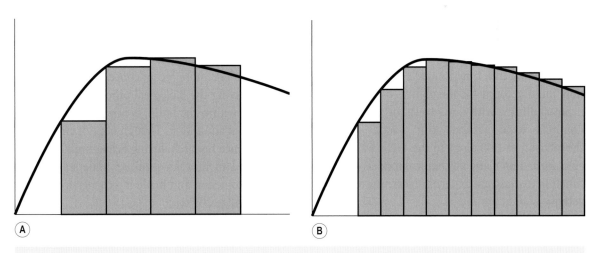

Figure 5.1
(A) Rectangles can be used to approximate the area under a curve. (B) When the rectangles become smaller in width, more can be used and the area under the curve can be approximated more accurately.

variables present in the body, brain, and nervous system. We exist in a state of constant flux, from stages of development to aging and atrophy, through synaptic formation and electrochemical processes, each affected by our experiences and connections with the outside world. Differentiation and integration in this context pertained to an ongoing process of breaking down, forming new connections, and adding all of the pieces together again, resulting in a reorganized whole. Through such a process, we could develop nuance and choice in our self-use, increasing our competencies and skill over a lifetime of unlimited learning.

Neurobiology and definitions of function in the human nervous system

At the beginning of the 1975 Feldenkrais/Pribram discussions, Pribram famously illustrated his concept of functional integration from the standpoint of neurobiology. He took a piece of chalk between his teeth and wrote "Feldenkrais" on the chalkboard, after which he began to discuss where Feldenkrais' conceptual knowledge and his own thinking outside the boundaries of traditional neuroscience merged. Pribram asked the audience to consider how traditional models of cortical function could account for the ability to write legibly, if not skillfully, with one's teeth, or toes, or non-dominant hand, without prior practice. Much of the focus in neurobiology in the 1970s was on synaptic formation using mechanical models of simple function to illustrate patterns of learning and brain activity.

In neurobiology, functional integration is the concept of a whole brain functioning as one. It describes the way in which thousands of neurons from each part of the brain, from lower to higher brain centers, between regions, and across hemispheres, become linked through electrochemical connections in response to stimulus (Hohwy 2007). Functional integration is behind the development of imaging from CT scanning to MRI, to current uses of fMRI to more directly study the way the nervous system processes information from the outside world. Interestingly, these models are now analyzed and studied using the differential equations of mathematics (Ermentrout 1998).

In biology, and indeed in brain development, differentiation is the process by which undifferentiated stem cells develop into cells of distinct function throughout an organism (Gilbert 2000). It is how a single cell develops into a multicellular organism, and it is how these cells give rise to various cellular structures and kinds of tissue that function to make a fully developed organism. To use another Feldenkrais term, a stem cell's "potency" describes the range of cells into which various stem cells are able to differentiate (Singh et al. 2016).

Feldenkrais' use of the term differentiation in the context of whole-brain functional integration applies to the increasingly fine and widespread variations of stimulus we can add to our experience to maximize these integrative connections throughout the brain. The more recent concept of neuroplasticity, involving the biological process of cell differentiation within the brain, is now known to occur throughout adulthood. Though not documented in neuroscience research during Feldenkrais' lifetime, he seemed to have an intuitive understanding of this phenomenon and made it a cornerstone of his work (Doidge 2015).

In sequences of motor development, Feldenkrais was also interested in how humans initially "differentiate" the use of muscles to perform the foundations of later motor function. Babies, for example, first contract all of the flexors and extensors at the same time; development and refinement of motor function involves making muscle groups and muscles themselves contract and de-contract independently (Feldenkrais 1975–1977, June 18). In terms of higher function and skill, Feldenkrais spoke interchangeably about the use of differentiation to create distinctions that break up habitual patterns and to avoid compulsive activity that stops us from further growth (Feldenkrais 1975–1977, June 19). These distinctions are made by using similar muscles and combinations of muscles and nerves in the context of multiple and varied intentions to act, or the differentiation of intent. He points out that we have only one set of each kind of muscle, such that any action that requires these muscles will involve the same structural contraction and de-contraction:

> There (are) only two biceps in the body, so any act in which a bicep has to be enrolled, like giving bread or money to someone, taking something from them, or pulling out a knife from someone's back, whatever the emotion, it's that bloody bicep that will have to perform it. The bicep will obviously get the order to contract from many different ideas; it can participate in all these different ways, with tension, anger, charity, goodness, etc. So, the integration in the nervous system is total but the main function with each of those contractions is in a different part of the brain. When it has to do with feeling, it comes from the thalamus; when it has to do with a different thing, it comes from the frontal lobe, but it's organized to learn from the motor cortex the achievement it can do and then relay it and give orders to the lower centers to perform it.
>
> Feldenkrais 1975–1977, July 2

A widely used example of this idea in Feldenkrais' *Awareness Through Movement* lessons involves the differentiation of the teleceptors, namely the eyes and the ears, from the function of the musculature of the head and neck, and other parts of the body (Feldenkrais 1975–1977, June 18). In some lessons

Feldenkrais explored differentiating the movement of the eyes from the turning of the head and the shoulders: keeping the head still while moving the eyes and the shoulders; moving the head independently while keeping the eyes fixed on one point; tracking the movement of each eye independently; and many other variations of this idea. In other lessons he included in- and out-of-phase movements of eyes and head with the movement of the pelvis, legs, and feet. In each variation he provided opportunities to discover new combinations of contractions and de-contractions in the musculature, and, more importantly, new intentions toward action in the world.

Evolution and phylogeny

In several of his discussions, Feldenkrais uses an example from the 20th-century French physician René Leriche to illustrate "differentiation" between high brain, or learned, and low brain, or phylogenetically inherited, responses (Feldenkrais 1975–1977, July 4). Leriche was one of the first researchers to theorize that certain kinds of physical trauma could be elicited purely due to inherited evolutionary traits originally adopted to protect us in situations of mortal danger. Leriche observed a particular phenomenon in knee injuries that involved no initial tissue damage, yet yielded immediate swelling and muscle atrophy (Mohanty 1946). He created a technique using novocaine to dull sensation in a newly traumatized knee to trick the brain into perceiving that the knee had been stabilized and avoid triggering the phylogenetic response (Feldenkrais and Pribram 1975).

Many of Feldenkrais' ATM lessons involve evolutionary themes and explore differentiation between higher brain function and lower phylogenetic protective responses. These may be found particularly in dealing with:

- extensor contraction in response to falling (anti-gravity)

- variation in functions and structures of breathing

- developmental moves – from lying, to rolling, to crawling

- exploring stages of movement representative of a kind of evolutionary progression from our life in water, to being on the land on all fours, to our current bipedal state.

The term "differentiation" as it is defined in evolutionary studies, similar to its use in neurobiology, refers to stem cell differentiation into various kinds of tissue to perform unique functions in the body, brain, and nervous system. This definition of cellular differentiation was important in Feldenkrais' thinking about evolution as well. Feldenkrais and Pribram together discussed ways in which lower and higher parts of the brain have become networked to meet new functional demands. For example, the cerebellum and the brainstem can network with parts of the cortex, parts of the brain which were long thought to only function independently of each other, enabling us to have control over certain autonomic processes (Feldenkrais and Pribram 1975).

Feldenkrais was fascinated by human evolution toward higher and higher levels of achievement, and the ability of each new generation to surpass the previous in discoveries, feats, and skills (Feldenkrais 1985). He illustrated his points through the work of scientists like Newton, Einstein, and, indeed, Leriche, as well as through the dramatic breaking of world records in sports and through new levels of artistic achievement in the most accomplished musicians and dancers (Feldenkrais 1975). Feldenkrais viewed these endeavors that repeatedly brought our species to higher thresholds of function as proof of the infinite capacity and competency of the human brain.

In the study of phylogeny and evolution, the term "phenotypic integration" describes the process by which groups of cells in multicellular organisms work together to perform a function (Pigliucci 2003). The more evolved a system is, the larger the variety of traits involved in each function. For example, at the lowest level of evolution, single-celled organisms are limited to a single function, such as reproduction, whereas, at the higher levels of multicellularity, groups of cells might integrate for the function of digestion or circulation. In complex organisms, these cells group to form complex systems, like the human brain and nervous system, and, indeed, brains and nervous systems which perform multiple functions, making them increasingly adaptable. Humans, being the most evolved multicellular organisms, are also the most functionally integrated phylogenetically, able to perform multiple functions and multiple variations of these functions. As Pribram demonstrated in writing with his teeth, and as Feldenkrais often said, an important result of evolution is the ability to meet a situation never before encountered with a response not specifically learned but, rather, spontaneously produced, derived from all past learning and phylogeny.

Psychology, learning, and human potential

Feldenkrais developed the concept of cognitive integration of movement, sensation, emotion, and thought. In the book *Awareness Through Movement,* he described these four elements of the "waking" state as the primary for all learning. He says that differentiated movement when applied with "awareness," a level of consciousness even higher than wakefulness, could induce an integration, or reorganization of each of these states by breaking down patterns of compulsion or habit (Feldenkrais 1972, p. 31, 39). He states in the chapter, "Where to Begin and How":

A fundamental change in the motor basis within any single integration pattern will break up the cohesion of the whole and thereby leave thought and feeling without anchorage in the patterns of their established routines. In this condition it is much easier to effect changes in thinking and feeling, for the muscular part through which thinking and feeling reach our awareness has changed and no longer expresses the patterns previously familiar to us. Habit has lost its chief support, that of the muscles, and has become more amenable to change.

Feldenkrais 1972, p. 39

In changing the patterns of habit and achieving higher levels of integration, we gradually free ourselves from the parasitic and contradictory patterns that create or inhibit our freedom of choice, intention, and action. For Feldenkrais, this ability to do what we want, to act with spontaneity, and to inhibit our actions only by conscious choices, epitomized maturity and potency in human behavior, the topic of his final book, *The Potent Self* (Feldenkrais 1985).

In 19th- and 20th-century studies in psychology and cognition, specific definitions of "integration" might be likened to Feldenkrais' descriptions of potency in human behavior, particularly theories and practice of the classic psychoanalysis of Adler and Jung (Feldenkrais 1949). Integration in psychology refers to the processes of maturation as a person becomes aware of and attentive to individual needs while functioning in a balanced relationship within his or her environment and society. In the earliest stages of human life we are entirely at the mercy of our individual needs for attention, sustenance, safety, etc. As we develop, we gain awareness of our surroundings and become functioning

members of society, but we also find ways of caring for ourselves individually and developing individual autonomy. Being well-integrated means that we maintain balance between self and other into and throughout adulthood. The concept of integration as a product of awareness and attention is common in many analytical systems and even religions directed at "correction" of compulsion. Feldenkrais referenced a variety of approaches to behavioral correction, from Freud and Coué (psychoanalysis and hypnotherapy), to Zen Buddhism and eastern practices of yoga, to aspects of Judaism and other dominant religions (Feldenkrais 1972).

In *The Potent Self* Feldenkrais expands on the idea of using differentiated movement to induce change in the integration of thought and emotion, thus demonstrating how his work could enhance the efficacy of other forms of psychotherapy which attempt to reorganize or correct by treating the psyche alone. He believed that habit formation and compulsion could be observed in movement with much more clarity than in thought or emotion. Furthermore, he believed that by exploring movement in finer differentiations, we can improve the balance between action and return to homeostasis in the nervous system (Feldenkrais 1985, p. 4). The introduction of more differentiated patterns of movement allows greater fluidity in action while assisting in the dissolution of previously dominating habits of emotion and thought, opening the doors to spontaneity, creativity, and achievement.

Further thoughts

As a musician, and teacher, I have found Feldenkrais' use of language and his keen semiotic sense as much of a tool for learning and application to my thinking and teaching as the many *Awareness Through Movement* lessons he left us. I am fascinated by the ways these ideas have led me outside the traditional boundaries of my own field of interest. There is an asymptotic process – one of continuously striving to parse, refine, and restructure in the pursuit of various ideals – that pervades Feldenkrais' discussion and writing that has entered my own work. Feldenkrais' process gradually reveals itself in the contents of his movement lessons through sensation, but it is a process that is complex enough that it would take years of doing these lessons over and over and exploring the myriad variations on individual themes, the changes in construction around similar themes, etc., to grasp even a fraction of the complexity of Feldenkrais' thought around these issues.

Feldenkrais' concepts of function, differentiation, and integration provide insights into human learning, development, evolution, and potency from various perspectives. They have helped me appreciate the complexity of learning, to think abstractly in developing my own theories into hypotheses, and they allow me additional freedom in thought and action. I hope as we continue to study and explore the work of Moshe Feldenkrais, we will find more questions and avenues for exploration and follow our founder's own example by broadening and deepening our work for many years to come.

References

Doidge, N. 2015. *The Brain's Way of Healing*. Viking, New York.

Ermentrout, G.B. 1998. *Differential Equations: Computational neuroscience*, self-published. University of Pittsburgh, Pittsburgh, PA.

Feldenkrais, M., Pribram, K. 1975. Introduction by Hanna, T., *Interview and Discussion*, sound recording by Hanna, T. San Francisco Feldenkrais Training.

Feldenkrais, M. 1949. *Body and Mature Behavior: A study of gravitation, anxiety, sex and learning*. International Universities Press, New York.

Feldenkrais, M. 1972. *Awareness Through Movement: Health exercises for personal growth*. Harper & Row, New York.

Feldenkrais, M. (transcribers unknown) 1975–1977. *San Francisco Feldenkrais Training Transcripts*. International Feldenkrais Federation, Paris.

Feldenkrais, M. 1985. *The Potent Self: A study of spontaneity and compulsion*. Frog Ltd/Somatic Resources, Berkeley, CA.

Gilbert, S.F. 2000. *Developmental Biology*, 6th edn. Sinauer Associates, Sunderland, MA.

Hohwy, J. 2007. Functional Integration and the Mind. *Synthese* 159(2):315–328.

Mohanty, J.K. 1946. Novocaine Infiltration in Acute Sprains. *The Indian Medical Gazette* 81(1):19–20. Available online: https://www.ncbi.nlm.nih.gov/pmc/articles/PMC5236165/?page=1 [Accessed June 24 2020]

Pigliucci, M. 2003. Phenotypic integration: studying the ecology and evolution of complex phenotypes. *Ecology Letters* (6)3: 265–272.

Reese, M. 2015. *Moshe Feldenkrais: A life in movement*, vol. I, pp. 67–69. ReeseKress Somatics Press, San Rafael, CA.

Singh, V., Saini, A., Kalsan, M., Kumar, N., Chandra, R. 2016. Describing the Stem Cell Potency: The various methods of functional assessment and in silico diagnostics. *Frontiers in Cell Biology* 4(134).

Stachel, J. 2001. *Einstein from B to Z*. Birkhauser, Boston, MA.

Other resources

Feldenkrais, M., Soloway, T., Baniel, A., Krauss, J. (eds.) 2013. *Alexander Yanai Lessons*. International Feldenkrais Federation, Paris.

Audiation *Awareness Through Movement* Audio Lesson taught by Lisa Burrell

It is an experience common to all Feldenkrais Method practitioners: to share the name of our practice with new people and then, on seeing puzzlement spread across their faces, feel the need to provide some context for the unfamiliar and, to many ears, unusual name. At this point there are many strategies.

"It is a form of somatic education," I have said, often to continued puzzlement.

"It is a kind of movement training focused on mind–body awareness." At least now I have avoided that troublesome word, *somatic*.

"It's a practice I teach people with Parkinson's disease to help them improve their balance and regain lost mobility." My conversation partner often visibly relaxes upon learning that I have a niche.

"It's a kind of movement practice that helped me with chronic pain issues stemming from a neck injury. Now I teach it to others in group classes and private sessions." Narrating my own story with the method has proven the most effective means of assuaging suspicion as to why I would be involved in this unknown quantity.

To these statements I have received a range of responses, often in the form of follow-up questions. I have been asked if Feldenkrais is a form of yoga or tai chi; whether it is related to mindfulness; whether it is a kind of massage or physical therapy. For some people, the information I offer about the Feldenkrais Method triggers a memory or an association, and they mention an experience that they or someone they know has had with the Alexander Technique, Hakomi or another somatic method, or type of body psychotherapy. Then they ask if it's *like that*.

For those of us who already know the deep pleasures and benefits of the Feldenkrais Method, constantly being asked to locate it in relation to other types of work can be tiring, if not exasperating. Upon reflection, however, I realize that not only is it more useful to offer sound and patient answers to these questions than to give them short shrift, but also that they are *good questions*. The Feldenkrais Method is not related to yoga or tai chi, but it is partially derived from judo. It is not a form of massage or physical therapy, but a significant percentage of Feldenkrais practitioners also do one or the other of those practices, and many massage therapists, physical therapists, and occupational therapists have been influenced by the Feldenkrais Method. And while the method has features that make it distinct from other somatic schools or body psychotherapies, it also has commonalities with all of them.

I bring up my experience of introducing the method to new audiences as a way of approaching this question: how do we locate where the Feldenkrais Method stands in relation to more mainstream aspects of Western culture? In a variation of Moshe Feldenkrais' well-known dictum, "If you know what you're doing, you can do what you want," I say, "If you know where you are, you can decide where you want to go."

As a historian, my favored way of assessing the location of the Feldenkrais Method has been to inquire into both its historical origins and those of somatic education at large. Entering this research rabbit hole as part of the PhD program in history at the University of Colorado, Boulder, I emerged – six years and many hundreds of pages later – with a dissertation on the topic. In this essay, I offer two lessons from the history of the Feldenkrais Method that I hope will be informative and also supportive of your efforts to learn about, practice, and/or teach it. Without further ado, these are:

1 The Feldenkrais Method is not a science (and shouldn't pretend to be one);

2 Practicing the Feldenkrais Method may result in spiritual experiences (or not).

The Feldenkrais Method is not a science (and shouldn't pretend to be one)

Lest I draw ire for saying that the Feldenkrais Method is not and should not pretend to be a science (a claim I extend to the field of somatics as a whole), let me add a parallel assertion: the field of medicine is not a science, and it also shouldn't pretend to be one.

In making these assertions, I am not saying that medicine or somatics should not be *informed* by science, but rather that they should not be *confused* with it. The latter is the province of scientism, the very commonplace practice of conflating the methods and findings of formal science with fields of activity that are more basically conditional, relational, and unpredictable. A simple example from medicine is the difference between, on the one hand, knowing that a certain drug or procedure has, on aggregate, been shown in scientific studies to be effective in treating a certain health problem and, on the other hand, discerning whether that drug or procedure should be recommended to the actual person in one's office. The former is statistical data derived from tightly regulated and controlled studies; the latter is a subjective decision that ideally takes into account a range of factors including the possibility of inaccurate diagnosis and the doctor's financial stake and other forms of potential personal or social bias, as well as the worldview, circumstances, and goals of the person who has come seeking help. Maintaining this distinction in practice has proven

to be one of the most vexing problems of contemporary Western medicine.

The distinction between scientific information and practice should be even clearer in the case of somatics. The two fundamental demands the scientific method makes upon a given claim are that it be public and replicable. (As a historian of science once said to me, "There is no *private* science.") By contrast, the Feldenkrais Method, like all somatic schools, tends to be much more concerned with the cultivation of personally useful and meaningful experiential knowledge.

This issue is perhaps trickier in the case of Feldenkrais than it is for most other somatic schools, because Moshe himself was an accomplished scientist. Initially self-taught, in the 1940s he earned a PhD in engineering at the Sorbonne under the guidance of Nobel laureate Frédéric Joliot-Curie. Moshe went on to work professionally as a scientist, doing research for the British Navy during World War II and then serving as head of electronic engineering for the army in newly formed Israel from 1951 to 1953. Even after he departed formal science to devote himself full time to developing and teaching his method, he often used scientific language when describing the theory behind it, its practice, and its results. He also remained in close contact with a number of scientists, including world-renowned figures such as Heinz von Foerster and Karl Pribram.

Given that Moshe was a successful scientist, why do I make such a fuss about distinguishing his method from science? To answer that, let me make an example: the notion that in practicing the Feldenkrais Method one rewires one's brain.

Moshe is rightly lauded for being ahead of his time in understanding the neuroplasticity of the adult brain. Although he was not a neurologist, he discerned from the neurological literature that every human action and experience has its correlate in the activity of the nervous system, which means that if we experience change, it must also be showing up as nerve activity. He often referred to the changeability of the brain in his teaching.

What we consider possible or impossible has nothing to do with reality because we behave like small babies having a huge brain and only using a small bit of it.

He said in a lesson from 1972. He continued:

And we wire it in such a way that the rest seems to us outside the range... Therefore, if you clear the brain of all this and allow it to function to its full power you will find that things that look absolutely impossible, out of human range, actually are within your easiest achievement.

Feldenkrais 2012, p. 229

Seeing this precedent in his claims and his languaging of the method, it is not surprising to find many Feldenkrais Method practitioners speaking of how it can rewire the brain. But neuroscience has changed quite a bit since Moshe's day. It's now widely assumed that the brain and nervous system are in a constant state of activity – either maintaining homeostasis or adapting to new conditions. In a certain sense, rewiring is just what the brain does. So what, precisely, do we mean when we claim that

the Feldenkrais Method *causes* rewiring? And how could we prove that it does?

In one sense, saying that the practice of Feldenkrais causes rewiring of the brain is a hypothesis that, phrased more explicitly, would be more like this: If you practice the Feldenkrais Method, you will sense noticeable differences in your experience, and we are quite sure that, if we were to put your brain into an imaging machine at the right time, these differences could be detected neurologically.

My own perspective is that, when we tell someone that the method can rewire their brain or nervous system, we are actually employing an analogy. We are saying, in effect, "Practicing this method can lead to such noticeable improvements in your experience that you will *feel as if* your brain has been rewired." This strikes me as a much more accurate way to view statements from Moshe such as those above, wherein he suggests that his students "clear the brain" of its faulty wiring and "allow it to function to its full power." How could one possibly check on such developments?

Why would a science-y analogy be more comforting and convincing to many people than simply hearing that they will experience positive change that

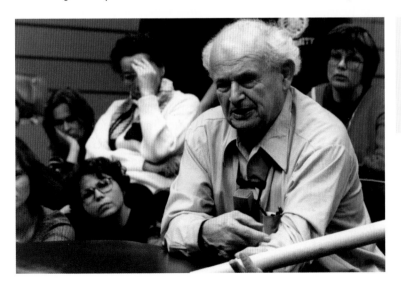

Figure 6.1
Moshe Feldenkrais teaching in Freiburg.

they can verify themselves? I'll give a very condensed version of my own opinion: I think this preference reflects the modern adaptation of that old bugaboo of Western materialism, the Cartesian dualism. No longer Descartes' originally postulated soul/body dichotomy but rather a brain/body dichotomy that assumes all meaningful change must originate in the brain. Even more directly: we simply live in a very scientistic culture, currently in a long-term fad wherein people love hearing mention of the brain. In other cultures, with other conceptual systems and values, we might instead be focused on the bodily humors, the heart-mind, the *hara*, or the *qi*.

Moshe was not the only founder of a somatic school to claim scientific validity for his or her method. F.M. Alexander (1869–1955), founder of the Alexander Technique, represented his work as a kind of scientific psychophysical laboratory for the individual. In this he had the strong backing of John Dewey, considered in his day to be one of the world's eminent scientific minds. Mabel Todd (1880–1956), the founder of a somatic school that came to be known as Ideokinesis, also consistently presented her work in a scientific frame. Indeed, given that most of the major lineages of somatic practice appeared between the 1890s and the 1950s, a timeframe in which science experienced an incredible ascent in intellectual and cultural prestige, it is not surprising that the founders of these methods sought to associate their work with science.

Crucially, however, these founders' scientific outlooks were formed in an era in which it seemed plausible that science might prove to be humanity's salvation. The late Feldenkrais Method Trainer Mark Reese addresses this point in his masterful biography of Moshe Feldenkrais:

Great idealism accompanied science in those times, and a sometimes utopian world-view. The prospect of a rational mastery of nature also brought the promise

of a more rational human order. Feldenkrais' own social values reflected this outlook... The miseries of World War I and the Great Depression strengthened the general sense that scientific principles should play a more decisive role in human affairs.

Reese 2015, p. 161

The clearest example of such idealism that I came across in my research on the history of somatics was that of evolution. Alexander, Todd, and Feldenkrais each espoused forms of progressive evolutionism, meaning the possibility of human evolution toward a higher state. This stands in contrast to Darwinian theory, which posits no particular goal, and in fact little in the way of directedness, in the process of evolution. The Darwinian view of evolution assumes that even an adaptation that supports a given species to thrive for a certain time may lead to its extinction as soon as environmental or climatic conditions change. Alexander, who did not have a firm grasp of Darwinian theory, was the most grandiose of the three, claiming that the spread of his method could lead to evolutionary advance not only for individuals but also for societies, races, and perhaps humanity as a whole. (This is apparent, for instance, in the subtitle of his first book: *Man's Supreme Inheritance: Conscious guidance and control in relation to human evolution in civilization*.)

Todd had a better understanding of Darwinian evolution, but she too allowed her evolutionism to extend beyond Darwinian boundaries to the possibility of the progressive improvement of humankind. For instance, she wrote, "In this mechanism [awareness and control of conditioned reflexes] lies the hope of further evolution and a higher civilization, the possibility of an integration of the spiritual values with factual education" (Todd 1978, p. 49). Concerning Feldenkrais himself, I again defer to Reese:

Moshe was drawn to 'progressive' conceptions of evolution that extended beyond Darwin's parameters. Francisco Varela commented that Feldenkrais had a utopian view of biology... Moshe's evolutionary orientation was not religious, but neither was it reducible to science. Moshe's evolutionary orientation was, true to his entire method, experientially based.

Reese 2015, p. 441

Looking at evolutionism in the work of Alexander, Todd, and Feldenkrais draws out a crucial point concerning the formation of somatics, which is that although it was related to science from the beginning, it was a profoundly syncretic field, including in its use of scientific information. The founders of these somatic schools wanted their work to encompass the lessons of Darwinian evolution *and more*. This could be said of the relationship between somatic education and other areas of science as well – physiology and more; developmental biology and more. Sometimes these founders spoke as if their work moved *from* science *to* experience, but when they did so they had succumbed to the temptation of scientism. The *and more* was the core of somatics, and it is precisely what Reese points to in the quote above – it is the experiential basis, phenomenology, the centering of lived experience.

To center lived experience excludes certain possibilities. One cannot, for instance, sense that one's brain has been rewired, nor can one feel evolution in the Darwinian sense of that term. Both of these refer to processes that require the broad, exacting eye of formal science for their verification. One may, however, experience greater ease in lying on the floor, a softer chest, a lengthening of the spine, an opening of vision, an upwelling of vitality, a sense of friendliness. Indeed, one can experience an infinite variety of things regardless of whether they have much in the way of relationship to the scientific method. And at that, I believe we have reached the right juncture at which to pivot to this essay's second topic: spirituality.

Practicing the Feldenkrais Method may result in spiritual experiences (or not)

Perhaps you took note of Reese's statement, quoted above, that "Moshe's evolutionary orientation was not religious, but neither was it reducible to science." I agree and am sure there's no controversy in saying more broadly that Moshe's work was not religious. He belonged to no religious sect or institution, and he enjoyed being iconoclastic toward religious figures and challenging toward any kind of religious dogmatism.

Yet there is also plenty of evidence that Moshe had a rich spiritual life that flowed into his articulation of the Feldenkrais Method. Both Reese (2015), in his biography of Moshe, and David Kaetz (2007), in his book exploring Moshe's Hasidic upbringing, have demonstrated strong connections between Moshe's teaching and Jewish mysticism. It's also clear that Feldenkrais understood judo in the way its founder, Jigoro Kano, intended it to be understood – as a holistic practice meant to engage the practitioner at all levels, including the spiritual. When naming *judo*, Kano chose the character *do* – the Japanese version of the *dao* in *Daoism*, meaning "way" in the East Asian sense of that word – to differentiate it from the more instrumental *jutsu* in *jujutsu*. (The first character is the same in each case.) And it is well known that Feldenkrais studied and admired the work of Greek-Armenian teacher G.I. Gurdjieff (1866–1949), who was among the major innovators of 20th-century Western esotericism.[1]

---

1 "Esotericism" here refers to a field of study developed over recent decades, focused on related currents in the history of Western religion, philosophy, art, and science; see Hanegraaff 2013, pp. 1–3 (also p. 42 on Gurdjieff's role in modern Western esotericism).

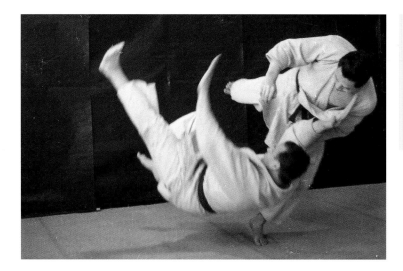

Figure 6.2
Judo Throw: Moshe Feldenkrais with Mikonosuke Kawaishi, who together founded the Jiu-Jitsu Club of France, 1938.

Hasidism, Japanese martial arts philosophy, and Gurdjieff's "Fourth Way" – these are an unusual blend of spiritual influences. While Moshe may have engaged the spiritual possibilities of the modern era with particular *chutzpah*, he was entirely normal in his access to so many sources of spirituality. Here, I use the word spirituality to indicate the practices and experiences of people who embrace secularism as an opportunity for creative blending. Many people, then and now, still maintain traditional religious affiliations, identifying themselves as Roman Catholics, Southern Baptists, Sunni Muslims, Orthodox Jews, Theravadan Buddhists, etc. What I mean by secularism, however, is that, whatever one's personal belief system, we live in an era where the majority of people in the world are unavoidably confronted with people who have different religious beliefs, including all varieties of agnosticism and atheism.

The proliferation of interreligious knowledge and encounter has been gathering steam for centuries, with no end in sight. In this sense, a conservative evangelical is as much living in a secular era as any New Age hippie or hardcore atheist. So, too, is any practitioner of the Feldenkrais Method or any other somatic school. And in this, I see a certain kind of symmetry with my earlier argument about science. Whereas formal science has undergone a narrowing of definition and methodology that has made it largely inhospitable to somatic worldviews and practices, spirituality has become so diffuse as to be virtually individual. Here, then, I come to the second thesis of this essay: practicing the Feldenkrais Method may result in spiritual experiences (or not).

Allow me first to address the "or not." The secular era easily encompasses non-spirituality, whether that means materialist atheism or simple denial that there is a spiritual dimension to one's existence. In a way that was not possible for much of human history – not possible, for instance, in the context of Moshe's childhood in Jewish *shtetls* in Eastern Europe – it is now possible to live without orientation to any kind of religious or spiritual practice.

At the same time, we are now perfectly free to choose such orientations, or to happen into them in ways that were far less likely in the more culturally bounded communities of earlier eras – like when Moshe happened across Jigoro Kano in Paris in the 1930s. Following this line of thought, I am led to the question: What might happen when a person begins to do a practice, such as the Feldenkrais Method, that supports a holistic inquiry into their thinking, emoting, sensing, and moving? In other words, what happens when a person begins a practice that invites awareness into all facets of their being? To answer this question, I will borrow a perspective from Buddhism. If someone undertakes non-instrumental awareness practice – that is, practicing an awareness discipline open-endedly and for its own sake – then, if they are not having spiritual experiences already, they are mightily susceptible to starting to have them. Let me set aside the word "spiritual," in case that's tripping anyone up, and continue by saying: they are susceptible to experiences of awe at the profoundly intricate and interrelated functioning of their body, mind, and environment. They are susceptible to experiences of wonder at the ineffable awareness that seems to be both already present and subject to discovery.

I will end by considering a quote from Moshe – the same quote, in fact, that I used earlier in referencing his views on rewiring the brain. It is from the series he taught at Esalen in 1972, from the lesson "Fingertips Under Armpits." He had just shown that a movement the students took to be impossible could be learned relatively quickly.

I have a whole series of things like that, showing that we don't really know how our spirit, our lamentation, how it works; what we avoid. What we consider possible or impossible has nothing to do with reality because we behave like small babies having a huge brain and only using a small bit of it. And we wire it in such a way that the rest seems to us outside the range.

Feldenkrais 1972, p. 229

Spirit and lamentation; the wiring of the brain. More soon followed: regarding the undoing of emotional patterns and always having choice. Moshe

was a brilliant individual, in fact a genius in many people's estimation. This small sample of his teaching is representative with regard to its audacious mix of perspectives and the boldness of its claims.

I hope that, in this essay, I have shown that the legacy of this brilliant but oftentimes inscrutable teacher can be fruitfully approached from the standpoint of historical analysis. Such analysis has led me to conclude that some of Moshe's opinions about the relationship between his method and science, though at home in his era, have grown out of sync with mainstream science. Moshe's take on evolution or on rewiring the brain may be useful as tools to help boost people's confidence in the method, but they also come with the risk of slipping into scientism.

Situating the Feldenkrais Method in a broader history of religion and spirituality has led me to conclude that, in the globalist field that is modern spirituality, this method, with its blend of religious influences and its invitation to holistic embodiment, is as well suited a player as any.

References

Feldenkrais, M. 2012. *Esalen 1972 Workshop: Awareness Through Movement lessons.* Feldenkrais Resources, San Diego, CA.

Hanegraaff, W.J. 2013. *Western Esotericism: A guide for the perplexed.* Bloomsbury Academic, New York.

Kaetz, D. 2007. *Making Connections: Roots and resonance in the life and teachings of Moshe Feldenkrais.* River Centre Publishing, Hornby Island, Canada.

Reese, M. 2015. *Moshe Feldenkrais: A life in movement.* ReeseKress Somatics Press, San Rafael, CA.

Todd, M.E. 1978. *Hidden You: What you are and what to do about it.* Reprint. Princeton Book Company, New York.

Zepelin, M. 2018. "From Esotericism to Somatics: A history of mind-body theory and practice across the divide of Modernism, 1820s to 1950s," PhD dissertation, University of Colorado, Boulder, CO.

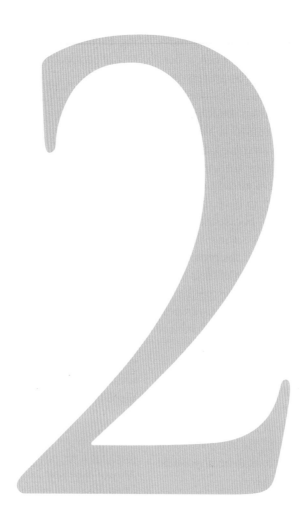

Beginning and pioneering

I could begin by saying that Dr Moshe Feldenkrais was a martial artist, not just in his youth, but also later on when he was developing, teaching, and promoting his method of *Awareness Through Movement*. He was more than that, though; Moshe was a Budoka – a man who walked the warrior's path and whose deep knowledge and experience of the martial arts led him to develop the Feldenkrais Method.

I am honored to write this chapter, sharing what I have learned as a researcher, martial artist, and Feldenkrais practitioner. My writing is based on research carried out over a period of 10 years, when I was investigating the synergy of the Feldenkrais Method and the martial arts.

Feldenkrais' life intersected with the martial arts at two major points. First, he joined the Haganah (a Zionist military organization representing the majority of Jews in Palestine from 1920 to 1948) at its inception in 1920, and in 1921 he began jiu-jitsu training with his fellow Haganah fighters. Second, in 1933 he entered the world of judo after meeting with Professor Jigoro Kano, the founder of modern judo, in Paris. He continued his involvement with the art in England until he returned to the State of Israel in 1950.

Black belt: what does it mean?

Moshe was one of the first people in Europe to receive a black belt in Judo. Today there are millions of people who have achieved this level, each with their own personal story. So what makes Moshe's achievement unique?

Moshe received his black belt in 1936. Considering that there were perhaps only a hundred black belts in Europe in the 1940s and 1950s, being among the first was indeed exceptional. In 1948, at the peak of his activity as a judoka, he was chosen to be the first non-European member of the judoka Council of the European Judo Union. As the chairman, T.P. Leggett, pointed out, "the purpose of the Council was not to represent national interest, but to be composed of real Judo experts."

Minimum effort, maximum efficiency

I had the good fortune to learn from two extraordinary Feldenkrais trainers, Carl Ginsberg and Dennis Leri. Leri wrote in his foreword to the reprinted *Higher Judo* (Feldenkrais 2010a), "Judo guided Moshe Feldenkrais' personal and professional research, and later formed the basis of the generalized system of learning that bears his name, the Feldenkrais Method."

In his foreword to the 2005 reprint of Feldenkrais' *Body and Mature Behavior*, Dr Carl Ginsberg wrote: "It was the study of self-defense, however, that was instrumental in setting his life's direction. Meeting Jigoro Kano, the founder of modern Judo, influenced him deeply."

In order to be "guided" and "influenced," one must be open to learning and able to change one's mind and one's body. Moshe was captivated by Kano and judo; equally amazing is the change in mind and body use that Moshe achieved through his own study of judo.

He began to move more like a judoka, adopting Kano's way of minimum effort and maximum efficiency. This change in Moshe's way of moving marked his evolution toward developing the

Feldenkrais Method. In fact, I maintain that his meeting with Kano on September 29, 1933, is a critical date in the Feldenkrais Method.

In 2013, when I interviewed Professor Harry Lipkin, a retired nuclear physicist who had worked under Moshe in the science division of the Israeli Defense Forces (IDF) in the early 1950s, the first words he said to me were, "Feldenkrais was ahead of his time and he is still ahead of his time." As the 91-year-old pointed out, "Feldenkrais knew a lot about physiology, judo, and electronics, and he combined this knowledge – a thing that no one else did at that time." The two men had often discussed Feldenkrais' ideas about how to cure people, and Lipkin understood how central judo was to the development of the Feldenkrais Method.

Bi-directional influence

My research also revealed that Moshe's "Feldenkraisian" thinking enriched his judo. I based my research on the assumption that judo had a significant influence on the Feldenkrais Method. Today I believe that the Feldenkrais Method formed Moshe's unique approach and way of teaching judo.

My research focuses on the years 1920–1950 that chronicle his path as a survivor and a fighter. These years provide us with solid facts and the fascinating story of his 30-year journey of Bu-Do (the Martial Way) – or "Moshe-Dō" (Moshe's Way).

Moshe showed mature wisdom, responsibility, and sensibility early in his childhood and youth, and it is notable that his way as a martial artist is characterized by his striving toward practicality and courage.

His warrior spirit, as well as his loyalty, were evident in a 1915 diary entry when he was 11 years old. Titled the "The City Garden!" he recounts how he chased a man who had stolen a hat from his friend and was making his getaway on a bicycle. The young Moshe dropped the perpetrator to the ground and recovered his friend's hat.

Moshe's courage and determination are further revealed when he traveled alone from his home in Russia to Palestine, aged 14, where he lived as a pioneer in poverty and danger. He began work there with his Baranovich group, constructing the city of Tel Aviv (Figure 7.1).

The following testimony by Avigdor Grünspan, a teacher turned laborer in Tel Aviv, is enlightening:

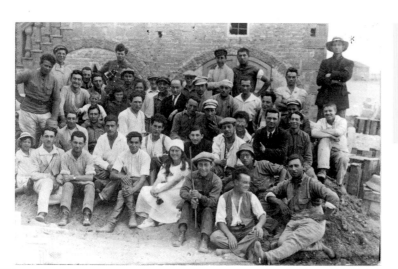

Figure 7.1
Moshe Feldenkrais (standing on the left), aged 16, with the Baranovich group, Tel Aviv, 1920.

Courtesy of Haganah Museum Archive, Tel Aviv

1920–1921:	Joined the Haganah and began Jiu-Jitsu training
1929–1930:	Translated Émile Coué's *Autosuggestion* and published *Jiu-Jitsu and Self Defense* for the Haganah
1933:	Met Professor Jigoro Kano in Paris
1934–1938:	Studied judo and published *A.B.C. du Judo*
1941:	Published *Judo: – The Art of Defence and Attack* in England
1942:	Published *Practical Unarmed Combat,* a training manual for soldiers
1947–1948:	Wrote *Higher Judo* (published 1952), *Body and Mature Behavior* (published 1949) and *The Potent Self* (published 1985)
1948–1949:	Wrote "Better Judo", a series published in the *Budokwai Bulletin*
1950:	Wrote his last, unfinished contribution for the *Budokwai Bulletin*, "Judo Research Work at the Budokwai"

Table 7.1 The milestones of Moshe-Dō show how thoroughly he was engaged with the martial arts.

My teacher on the site was a former pupil of mine named Moshe Feldenkrais. He was a young boy, around 16 years, broad-shouldered and sturdy as an oak.

Feldenkrais assigned me the task of climbing up to the second story of the building with him, carrying pallets full of cement and heavy stones.

Feldenkrais paid no attention to my groans and urged me to climb. "Make an effort, Grünspan," he said. "Pay no attention to the suffering: the Torah drains your strength, not the work; the work makes life sweet."

When I entreated him not to hurry so, he answered: "You are my spiritual teacher and I listen to you and obey you. I, however, am your material teacher and therefore you must obey me! You will eventually see that I am right."

Moshe's jiu-jitsu

When Moshe joined the Haganah in 1920 he fought under combat conditions alongside his friends. The rules of engagement on this battlefield were determined by the circumstances of the pioneers in the land of Israel in the period under the British Mandate, where Jews were not permitted firearms, so the weapons used were mostly knives, sticks, and barehanded techniques.

Although the Haganah fighters were trained in jiu-jitsu, they were not always able to make practical use of it in actual combat. Feldenkrais' friends were injured and even killed. He was troubled by these disappointing results, wondering why his friends could not use their skills to protect themselves more effectively. It was an opportunity for him to find a solution.

In 1930 Feldenkrais published *Jiu-Jitsu and Self-Defense*, a unique document showcasing his distinctive concept of survival and a systematic training regime (Figure 7.2). It was the first self-defense book written in Hebrew and marked the beginning of the development of Israeli self-defense systems, leading to the popular military Krav Maga system. The principles of learning and of fighting tricks make this early book an important document.

Just a year earlier Moshe had published his translation of *Autosuggestion* by Émile Coué, adding a monograph where he connected the unconscious to the conscious:

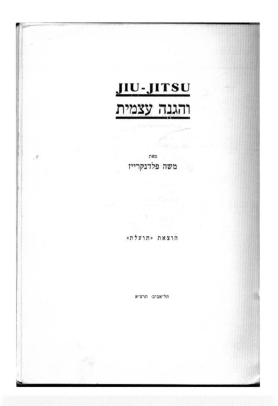

Figure 7.2
Cover pages of jiu-jitsu book.

Courtesy of Moti Nativ

The majority do not even know where exactly the solar plexus is, although the moment someone fears an attack directed towards themselves, they will unconsciously bend forward, and thereby defend this vulnerable place with their ribs... this defensive movement was fixed this way, and we will do it in spite of our conscious will.

Feldenkrais 2013, pp. 2–3

Feldenkrais designed a self-defense system based on a movement someone would do without thinking. The insight that inspired his method of self-defense was the opposite of the commonly held process of acquiring fighting skills. Usually we train so that the body reacts without thinking during an emergency. Moshe, however, showed the opposite path: first he investigated the unconscious or instinctive self-defense response (Figure 7.3). He maintained that it is easier and quicker to teach someone a new technique that is an extension of whatever they already do habitually. He believed that this approach would make it easy to perform efficiently in an emergency, even after a long break in training, because the *unconscious* reaction would arise spontaneously. He understood that natural movement is the foundation for faster learning. Dr Guy Mor, a Krav Maga expert,

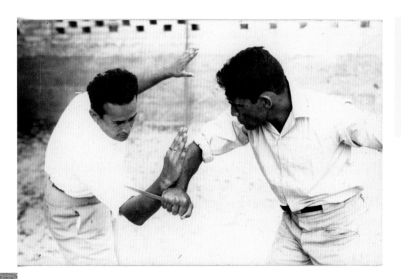

Figure 7.3
Instinctive defense against a knife stab by Moshe Feldenkrais, 1930.

published an academic paper in which he showed that Feldenkrais was the first person to train fighters using instinctive reactions as a springboard for effective combat and self-defense (Mor 2019).

Moshe opens the book *Jiu-Jitsu and Self-Defense* with the following words to the reader:

Remember, you will be stronger. To do good or evil will be in your hands. Please do not cause harm! Be careful, even with your enemies. I have labored so hard at this work not for the sake of war, but for Shalom (peace).

He justifies his book with the quote,

If I am not for myself, who then is for me?
Rabbi Hillel, 30 BCE–9 CE;
Feldenkrais 1930, pp. 8–9

Two significant things from this period are boxing and knife technique.

Feldenkrais learned boxing skills from his sparring partner Emil Avinery, a regional boxing champion, and soon became a great admirer of boxers and boxing. In the Feldenkrais training held in San Francisco, Moshe talked about the fight between Baer, a small-statured boxer, who beat Carnera, a large man.

He cited this fight as an example of the power of efficient movement: "… and there came Baer who was half his weight and made a mess of him. It's not a question of size; it's a question of the quality of action" (Feldenkrais, San Francisco Professional Training Program, Week 1, Day 1, June 16, 1975).

Later, at the Feldenkrais training in Amherst, Feldenkrais addressed concepts of efficient body manipulation through boxing. Demonstrating an elegant uppercut punch, he emphasized the correct organization of the skeleton:

The earth actually pushes me with the elastic forces of the floor at my foot, but when my skeleton, once it is organized so all the joints stand clearly one on top the other, not like that, not like this, not idiotically, then, the entire weight is annihilated by the elastic forces of the ground…
Feldenkrais, Amherst Professional
Training Program, June 30, 1980

In *Jiu-Jitsu and Self Defense*, Moshe presented a unique technique for defending against a knife stab using only one hand (Figure 7.4). He demonstrated this technique during his meeting with Kano. Later he wrote about the knife technique in his book,

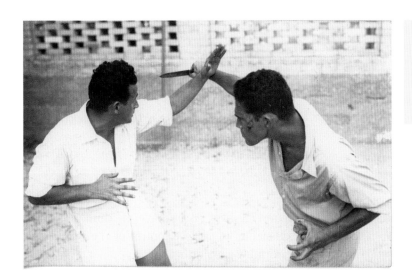

Figure 7.4
Knife technique (Moshe on the *left*).

A.B.C. du Judo (1938), and demonstrated it in the San Francisco training.

Entering the world of judo

Feldenkrais' Jiu-Jitsu book was the catalyst for his meeting with Professor Jigoro Kano. The 72-year-old Kano's abilities astonished Moshe. Kano wrote about this meeting in his diary:

I grabbed him in a tight reverse cross with both hands and said, "Try to get out of this!" He pushed my throat with his fist with all his might. He was quite strong, so my throat was in some pain, but I pressed on his carotid arteries on both sides with both hands so the blood could not get to his head, and he gave up.

Kano 2005, p. 49

The conceptual and physical changes that followed this meeting indicated a clear turn on his path toward the creation of the Feldenkrais Method. With Kano's support, he immersed himself not only in studying judo but also in teaching and promoting it in France, where he earned the title *Pionnier du Judo*.

In *A.B.C. du Judo*, written in French just four years after he began to practice judo, he combines judo, self-defense, and physics. During this period, he had a meaningful connection with Mikonosuke Kawaishi, a high-level judoka. Feldenkrais trained with him in Paris and Kawaishi promoted him to second Dan. They photographed many techniques and Moshe used the photos in both his *Judo* and *Higher Judo* books.

Judo: The art of defence and attack (1941)

When the Nazis invaded France in 1940, Moshe escaped to the UK, where he found a new opportunity for judo. While posted as a scientist to a submarine base in Scotland, he published *Judo: The art of defence and attack*, in which he guides the student in learning judo techniques and how to apply them for more effective street fighting.

We get the sense that the seeds of the Feldenkrais Method were already germinating. For instance, "In Judo, the body is educated to respond faithfully and implement *the mental image* of the desired act" (Feldenkrais 1941, p. 12). This fits the logic of the famous introductory sentence in his book *Awareness through Movement*, "We act in accordance with our self-image" (Feldenkrais 1972, Preface).

Another significant principle of judo training is the improvement of "the senses of time and space" (p. 11). This refers to orientation, which is about movement in time and space. As he noted in *Mind and Body*, "The most important rule to observe in practice is to attend to manipulation and orientation in their widest meaning, at all times" (Feldenkrais 2010b, Conclusion).

Moshe enthusiastically describes practicing judo:

It is planned to improve general well-being... and develops coordination of movement as no other method or sport can possibly do... Indeed, judo should be considered as a basic culture of the body... invaluable preliminary to such artistic professions as dancing or acting, as well as to any sport or occupation where physical fitness and grace of movement are essential.

Feldenkrais 1941, pp. 11–12

He indicates,

For constant attention is paid in Judo, simultaneously with the teaching of attack and defense in the most efficient way, to the paramount aim of enabling men and women to have perfect control over mind and body.

p. 14

Figure 7.5 gives an example of Moshe's detailed explanation of perfect control of the body while performing a hip throw.

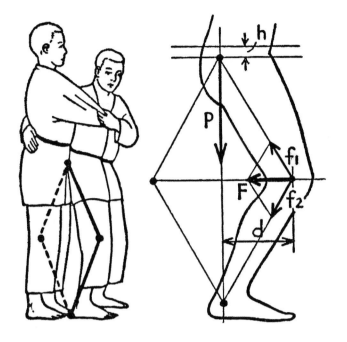

Figure 7.5
Hip throw.

Drawn by Moshe Feldenkrais

Practical Unarmed Combat (1942)

During Moshe's service in Scotland in World War II, the commander of a Home Guard platoon approached him and challenged him to teach his men unarmed combat. Moshe embraced this opportunity to test in practice the soundness of his unique scheme: confining learning to one technique. Hadaka Jime ("naked hands choke", Figure 7.6), paradoxically creates options, and options always provide more freedom of action.

Moshe linked this learning to unconscious action: "The ultimate value of an exercise lies in the action

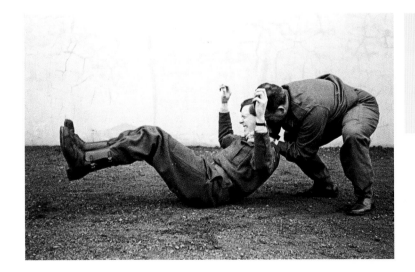

Figure 7.6
Hadaka Jime (Naked Hands choke; Moshe Feldenkrais on the *right*).

© International *Feldenkrais*® Federation, Paris, France. All rights reserved your body will perform spontaneously, without conscious effort, long after you have forgotten how, when, and where you have learned it" (Feldenkrais 1942, p. 15).

The training that he developed for the soldiers became a practical manual that everyone can use. "I devised this emergency course. It provides 'first-aid' equipment" (p. 14). Moshe designed a speedy way to instruct soldiers in self-defense through learning principles and techniques. The result was encouraging, and in a few months almost the entire battalion was trained.

Higher Judo (1952)

Moshe Feldenkrais' book *Higher Judo: Groundwork* represents a turning point in his life, written at the end of a period of intensive activity as a judoka.

The ideas expounded in the first four chapters could easily be taken for Feldenkrais' early writings about his method. This connection becomes obvious when you consider the fact that Feldenkrais was working on *Higher Judo* concurrently with *Body*

and Mature Behavior (1949) and *The Potent Self* (not published until 1985), which were all written between 1946 and 1948.

Higher Judo is a book that contains a unique presentation about the essence of judo. It includes detailed explanations about ground techniques that Moshe learned in 1938 while training with Mikono-suke Kawaishi (Figure 7.7).

Gunji Koizumi's original foreword to *Higher Judo* tells of his great appreciation of the book, of Moshe's wisdom, and his contribution to judo:

Such a study has been long awaited and is a very valuable contribution to a fuller understanding and appreciation of the merits of judo. Dr Feldenkrais, with his learned mind, keen observation and masterly command of words, clarifies the interrelation and the intermingled working of gravitation, body, bones, muscles, nerves, consciousness, subconscious and unconscious, and opens the way for better understanding.
Koizumi's Foreword, Feldenkrais 1952, pp. vii–viii

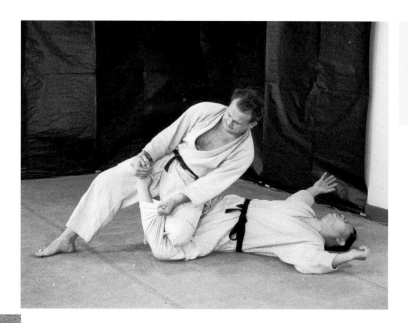

Figure 7.7
Feldenkrais and Kawaishi "breaking" knees.

Moshe's words on the objectives of judo can also be applied to the objectives of the Feldenkrais Method:

The essential aim of Judo is to teach, help and forward adult maturity... an ideal state rarely reached, where a person is capable of dealing with the immediate present task before him without being hindered by earlier formed habits of thought or attitude.

Introduction, pp. xii–xiii

Is Moshe talking about judo or about the Feldenkrais Method here?

Furthering the development of any function of the body that became habitually fixed restores harmonious growth of personality. For not only does the inhibited function become operative sooner or later, but the centers engaged in inhibiting the others are freed and become active in the expanding personality. The vitality of the whole organism is increased and a new interest in life appears. Such transformations are often produced by psychiatric treatment, when the complaint is so advanced that treatment is necessary. Judo, in expert hands, could be of considerable help in such cases. It is unique, however, in furthering normal growth towards adult independence in every normal person. And it does so by providing a highly pleasurable occupation at that. The beneficial effect is provided not as a medicine, but as another opportunity to learn to live fully.

pp. 40–41

"Better Judo"

Throughout a series of articles written and published for judo practitioners over the span of a year, we witness the integration of judo and the Feldenkrais Method. It closes with his suggestions to improve judo training by using five principles:

1 Make mistakes

2 Start learning with slow movements

3 Attain reversibility in action

4 Attain good posture for freedom of movement and breathing

5 Reduce effort to increase sensitivity.

Moshe guides the judoka according to the ideas and principles that we now know as the fundamental theories of the Feldenkrais Method.

Research

Moshe started writing his last and unfinished publication about judo for the *Budokwai Bulletin* in January 1950, "Judo Research Work at the Budokwai." He raised the concept of "transfer of learning," saying that "it is rather an elusive notion, which means the improvement of one kind of act by practicing another, such as the improvement of Hane-Goshi due to learning Harai-Goshi..." He states, "When viewed in its generality, transfer of training is the most important purpose of learning and training in general." Further, "The object of my investigation is to establish, if possible, the essential features of correct action, so as to be able to transfer the learning."

Thirty years later, he talked about the same concept:

... we are learning a process of organization so that all movements improve... therefore it is the quality that you learn in order that you can transfer... see whether you can actually transfer the learning. When I say get up and do something else, you do it with the same organization.

Feldenkrais, Amherst Professional
Training Program, July 7, 1980

The question that began the research into judo in 1950 is answered by the Feldenkrais Method.

Moshe and the martial arts after 1950

The supposed end of Moshe-Dō was when Moshe returned to Israel in 1950 and was made the head of the electronic department in the science division of the Israeli Defense Force. Looking back on Moshe Feldenkrais' life, it is clear that the martial arts were an integral part of his life until 1950, after which he devoted himself to what we know as the Feldenkrais Method. However, true martial artists walk on the martial way all their lives and Moshe remained a martial artist until his last day of teaching. There are many examples of this.

For instance, in *The Master Moves* he states that "… you see that the question of good movement is primarily whether it assures your survival and

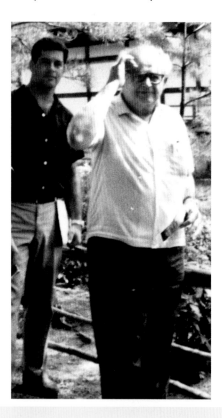

Figure 7.8
Moshe Feldenkrais and Danny Waxman in Tokyo, 1968.

Courtesy of Danny Waxman

self-preservation, and for that it is important to attend to propulsion" (Feldenkrais 1984, pp. 37–38). Slightly earlier, in the *Elusive Obvious* he writes, "The third biological criterion of posture… is self-preservation… self-preservation is the most stringent measure of good movement…" (Feldenkrais 1981, p. 50).

In 1968 Feldenkrais visited Japan. He was accompanied by Mia Segal (famous in her own right as a judoka and Feldenkrais trainer) as well as Gideon Kadari and Danny Waxman, two Israeli judo champions (Figure 7.8). Danny described how Feldenkrais entered the Kodokan and met Sumiyuki Kotani, a senior judoka and the chief instructor. Moshe reminded Kotani that he had met him in Paris in 1933, and that they had engaged in a long conversation, at the end of which Kotani had removed a special badge of honor pin from his own jacket and given it to him, something that Feldenkrais had always been very proud of.

In the Amherst training, Feldenkrais found many opportunities to teach like a martial artist. He showed how the power of the pinky fingers can break an opponent's balance; performed an accurate uppercut that lifted someone from sitting to standing; explained the power of a well-organized skeleton; and demonstrated a beautiful fencing movement (the "Errol Flynn" *Awareness Through Movement* lesson). He also demonstrated his famous knife technique. Moshe performed these techniques effortlessly, with the elegance and effectiveness of a high-level martial artist.

Summary

Many Feldenkrais practitioners don't know that Feldenkrais was a martial artist. That makes sense, because he taught the Feldenkrais Method and not the martial arts. But perhaps after reading this chapter, you will realize that as Moshe practiced and wrote about judo, he went through interesting processes of learning and development. These gave him personal and professional insights, which led him to investigate and formulate the fundamentals of the Feldenkrais Method.

As a Feldenkrais practitioner, there are times when I feel exhilarated after teaching a movement combination that seems like my own creation. However, I usually discover that Moshe had already taught it in his own way. For many years I was proud that my first *Awareness Through Movement* students were martial artists. But during the course of my research, I understood that even this Moshe had already done, because his first students were indeed the judokas.

I end this chapter with an example that raises and maybe answers the question: did judo influence the Feldenkrais Method or vice-versa? As Moshe stated at the beginning of his "Better Judo" series, "I prefer therefore, to present to you *another way of looking at things you already know...*" (Feldenkrais 1949).

Maybe it would be right to shift our perspective and say that judo influenced the development of the Feldenkrais Method. The facts show that Moshe developed as a martial artist *concurrent* with his development as a Feldenkrais practitioner.

Perhaps we should consider changing the name Feldenkrais Method to Feldenkrais Art.

I hope that this chapter will raise the awareness of Feldenkrais practitioners and other somatic practitioners and encourage you to share this information with your students. Moshe's uniqueness as a judoka should be acknowledged as the wellspring of the individualistic thinking that informed the development of the Feldenkrais Method.

References

Feldenkrais, M. 1930. *Jiu-Jitsu and Self-Defense* (Hebrew). Toellet, Tel Aviv.

Feldenkrais, M. 1941. *Judo: The art of defence and attack.* Frederick Warne, London.

Feldenkrais, M. 1942. *Practical Unarmed Combat.* Frederick Warne, London.

Feldenkrais, M. 1948–1949. Better Judo. *Judo Quarterly Bulletin*, vol. V, no. 4. The Budokwai: London.

Feldenkrais, M. 1952. *Higher Judo: Groundwork.* Frederick Warne, London.

Feldenkrais, M. 1975–1977. *San Francisco Feldenkrais Training Transcripts* (transcribers unknown). International Feldenkrais Federation, Paris.

Feldenkrais, M. 1981. *The Elusive Obvious.* Meta Publications, CA.

Feldenkrais, M. 1984. *The Master Moves.* Meta Publications, CA.

Feldenkrais, M. (1949) 2005. *Body and Mature Behavior: A study of anxiety, sex, gravitation, and learning.* Reprint. Frog Books, Berkeley, CA.

Feldenkrais, M. (1952) 2010a. *Higher Judo: Groundwork.* Reprint. Somatic Resources, San Diego, CA.

Feldenkrais, M. 2010b. Mind and Body. In: E. Beringer (ed.) *Embodied Wisdom: The collected papers of Moshe Feldenkrais*, pp. 27–44. North Atlantic Books, Berkeley, CA.

Feldenkrais, M. 2013. *Thinking and Doing.* Reprint. Genesis II Publishing, Longmont, CO.

Kano, J. 2005. *Mind Over Muscle: Writings from the founder of judo.* Translated by Nancy H. Ross. Kodansha International, Tokyo, Japan and Kodansha, America.

Mor, G. 2019. The Case for the Recognition of Krav Maga as Part of the Intangible Cultural Heritage of Israel. *Scientific Research* 7(4):294–303.

Other resources

Baer vs. Carnera boxing match 1934. www.youtube.com/watch?v=cf67JevtNcc

Erez, Y. 1964. *The Book of the Third Aliyah* (Hebrew). Am Oved Publishers Ltd., Tel Aviv.

Rolling the Fists and Transferring the Learning
Awareness Through Movement Video Lesson
taught by Moti Nativ
Courtesy of Kwan Wong, dailyimprovement.org

A child is born. It is a miracle. For the first few weeks, the little one sleeps a lot, nurses, occasionally cries, and needs to be held and rocked. Her arms and legs move, and her body twitches – all involuntary movements. Soon her family notices she is doing things she was unable to do before. When she is picked up, she holds her head up by herself. She reaches out to touch her mother's face. She clings to a parent's finger or a small toy. She rolls over by herself. By the time two years have passed, this little person can walk, talk, even argue, and she continues to grow, learn, and change at an incredible rate. Those around her expect, even assume, that she will eventually have a full, successful adult life, though no one knows what that will be.

As parents and caregivers, we look for ways to provide for the child's needs and do our best to give the child important support in her development. Yet, we have limited understanding of how the child's remarkable developmental changes come about. And we certainly have no direct control over when and how these changes actually occur.

When this magnificent, spontaneous process of development is disrupted due to cerebral palsy, autism, stroke, genetic anomalies, birth defects, ADHD, or other causes, we are faced with the challenge of finding ways in which we can help the child develop.

There are many educational and therapeutic approaches, each offering its own theories, methodologies, and levels of success. All share the goal of helping the child to overcome challenges and live a full and satisfying life.

The approach presented in this chapter, Anat Baniel Method NeuroMovement (an evolution from the Feldenkrais Method), is the science and practice of taking advantage of the brain's remarkable ability to change for the better through movement and touch, guided by the *Nine Essentials*," which I explain in some detail. This practice often makes the seemingly impossible possible, one step at a time.

Shoes out the window

I was sitting in my office on the 40th floor waiting for my new client, Max, to arrive. Max was a seven-year-old boy diagnosed with ADD/ADHD. He was struggling with learning math, reading and writing, and his teachers were complaining about his disruptive behaviors.

The door flew open and Max bolted into the room, scanned it briefly, then quickly took off his shoes. Holding one shoe in each hand, he ran toward a partially open window. His mother shouted, "Don't throw the shoes out the window, we just bought them!" Max, oblivious, continued straight toward the window.

I moved quickly and blocked his path as Max ran toward me. In a clear and calm voice, I asked, "Which shoe do you want to throw out first – the one in your right hand?", pointing at that hand, "Or the one in your left hand?" Max stopped abruptly and looked at me as though noticing me for the first time.

I repeated my question and Max looked at his hands, seeming to suddenly realize he was holding the shoes. I asked him to go over to his mom and give her the shoes, which he did. I then guided him to the treatment table, asked him to lie on his belly (which he did), and began working with him.

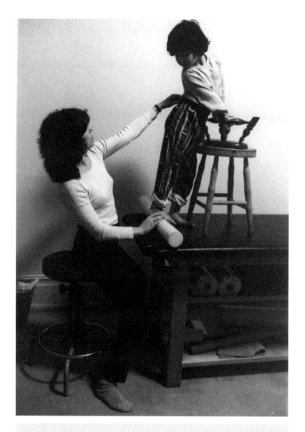

Figure 8.1
Anat Baniel working with a child.

Courtesy of Anat Baniel

Even though Max could walk, run, sit, etc., I wondered *how* he was doing these movements. How well was his brain *organizing* the movements he was doing? As he lay on his belly, I put my hand under one of his shoulders and gently lifted it up a little toward the ceiling. The whole of his back on that side lifted with his shoulder as if it were one unarticulated block, that is, as if there were no joints in there at all. What that indicated to me was that his brain was organizing this movement with very limited *differentiation*. Greater differentiation in the way the brain organizes the movements of all areas

of our body allows for new possibilities and learning to emerge (Prasad 1980, pp. 2–3; Mizrahi 2007). It also increases refinement, dexterity, complexity, and control in what we do (Wallace et al. 2017). What's more, greater differentiation in the brain is associated with enhanced cognitive abilities. Seeing the block-like movement of Max's back and shoulder, it was no wonder that math, reading, and writing were challenging for him. These cognitive skills require higher levels of differentiation and complexity than his brain had developed thus far.

I proceeded to move Max gently in a variety of ways. He lay there quietly, deeply attentive to feeling himself in new ways. His spine, ribs, shoulder blades, and pelvis began moving in new ways that were more differentiated, flexible, fluid, and harmonious. His breathing got fuller and there seemed a greater ease throughout his body. When I slowly helped Max off the table, he was quiet and peaceful.

Max returned for his next session two days later. His mom told me, with great excitement, that the teachers had noticed he was much calmer in class and doing better not only with math but even with reading and writing. "And we only had one session with you!" she exclaimed.

Too weak to move

The first time I saw Melinda, she was ten months old and reclining in an infant car seat. When her mother picked her up, her head fell forward and her body hung down from her mom's arms like a rag doll. I had never seen a child like her before.

Melinda's mom placed the car seat on the worktable. Although Melinda's body lay listless, she looked at me, alert and attentive. As I observed her, I noticed she did not move at all, except for her eyes and fingers. The latter she moved with exceptional levels of control, refinement, and dexterity for her age. How come, I wondered? Is something wrong with her brain? Or perhaps with the nerves connecting her brain to the rest of her body? Or is it something to do with her muscles?

Doctors had performed all the medical tests, including genetic testing, and could not determine a cause or a diagnosis for her condition. The mother told me Melinda had been getting therapy for a few months. When placed on her belly, she couldn't lift her head. When sat up, she needed to be fully supported or she would fall down. There were even unsuccessful attempts to make her stand up.

The way Melinda moved her eyes and fingers informed me that her brain was able to form highly differentiated and organized movements. Why, then, was she not moving the rest of her body? Then it dawned on me. Her tiny fingers were very light and required minimal effort to move. The same was true for her eyes. *The difference between the fingers and eyes and the rest of Melinda's body was weight.* When her brain sent signals to the muscles of her fingers or eyes to move, the muscular force required was small enough so that even with her very weak muscles, the neural signals resulted in movement. However, when her brain sent signals to the much heavier back, pelvis, head, legs, and arms, the muscles were too weak to move those parts. When the brain gets no response from the signals it sends out to the muscles and there is no movement, it eventually gives up: over time it sends fewer and fewer signals to those parts. Connections between these areas of the body and the brain are not formed. Without the representation of these areas in the brain – called "mapping" – the muscles have no opportunity to move and become stronger. Melinda's brain had only been able to map her eyes and fingers.

If I could find ways to help Melinda initiate movement, any movement that required no more force than it took for her to move her fingers and eyes, she could then *feel* herself moving and map those areas in her brain. Her brain could begin differentiating and forming the billions of neural connections required for her to learn to roll, sit, stand, and talk. We could then find out if those muscles would grow stronger, the way muscles usually do when we exercise.

I placed Melinda lying on her side and put a toy in front of her. She stared at the toy with great interest. Like any other baby, she wanted to reach out and touch it. When I saw her interest in the toy, I supported her arm, taking over most of its weight so that the arm, for her, became and felt very light. At the same time, I gently supported her spine. Her torso, which was shaped like a cylinder and required little effort to initiate movement, rolled forward. When her brain sent her arm signals to reach out and touch the toy, she easily accomplished this, even with her very weak muscles.

Melinda experienced, for the first time in her life, moving and successfully getting the outcome she was seeking.

Over time, Melinda grew stronger. First, when lying on her back, she began to lift her legs and arms and move them in the air, like babies typically do. She then learned to roll from her side to her belly, then from her back to her belly. In a few weeks, her back muscles became strong enough for her to fully lift her head up. Over time she learned to come up on all fours and crawl, then sit, and eventually stand up and walk.

It's important to note that I was not bound by the timeline of the typical "developmental stages." On the contrary, I made sure that any demands I placed on Melinda matched what she was able to do at that time. As she grew stronger, moving *spontaneously* in new ways, thanks to her developing more complex underlying neural networks, I presented her with configurations of movement that had not been available to her thus far. The brain of the typically developing child goes through the exact same process, though the trajectory and timeline may be quite different.

Trying to accelerate the child's development, as with "Tummy Time," bouncers, walkers or other techniques or devices, can interfere with the process of differentiation, impeding the creation of underlying neural networks from which new skills emerge and evolve. In a child with special challenges, such interference may even rob them of the ability to overcome their limitations (McEwan et al. 1991).

She got an "A" in math

Lizzi, aged ten, had been diagnosed with a severe scoliosis. The doctor recommended a brace to be applied right away, and if the brace didn't reduce the curvature, surgery would be required.

For the first month, Lizzi received a few private sessions a week combined with recorded Neuro-Movement lessons she did at home. Through these lessons the mobility in her back increased greatly. She joined the girls' basketball team and looked taller and straighter.

One day, four weeks into her program with us, Lizzi came for a session where her mother proudly announced that Lizzi had got an "A" in her latest math test. I responded mildly, "That's great!" Then her mom said: "Anat, you don't understand. Lizzi was failing in math and her work with you is the only new thing we have done. She is also a lot more socially active now."

The last time I saw Lizzi, the doctor cleared her from the need for a brace or surgery, and she proudly told me, "A lesson a day keeps the brace away."

What is the job of the brain?

Breakthroughs such as the ones that Max, Melinda, and Lizzi experienced start with asking this important question: what is the job of the brain? The brain does have a job to do, just like the heart has a job (to pump blood), the ears (to hear and maintain balance), and the muscles (to generate movement).

The job of the brain is to put order in the disorder and make sense out of the nonsense. The brain takes the vast and continuous flow of stimulation coming through our senses and organizes it into all that we require for living: our thoughts, our feelings, our emotions, our perceptions, our memories, our movements, our creativity, and all of our actions.

As a mechanical system that has mass, weight, and volume, our body adheres to the laws of Newtonian physics. For example, the heavier an object, the greater the force required to lift it. This is how we experience ourselves and the world from birth, and we expect, knowingly or unknowingly, for our brain to work according to the same mechanical rules.

The brain, however, works by very different laws. *It is an information system.* There isn't a mechanical force or lever that we can apply directly to the brain to make it work better. What the brain needs is stimulation, but stimulation alone is not enough. It is through the brain's ability to *perceive differences* in the flow of input from our senses that sheer chaos and a formless, meaningless sensory soup is transformed into clear perceptions and effective action.

When perceiving differences – what neuroscientists call signal-to-noise ratio – the brain differentiates through the growth of new connections and can spontaneously integrate some of these connections into new neural networks, thus forming new skills. This process is essential for successful learning.

The brain of the child with special needs is challenged in its ability to perceive differences for any number of reasons. The more we can help the brain of such a child improve in its ability to perceive differences in the flow of stimulation, the more information it will have for overcoming limitations. This is true irrespective of the diagnosis.

Visual demonstration of differentiation

1: Minimal differentiation

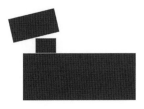

Figure 8.2
Minimal differentiation, 3 parts.

Look at Figure 8.2. What do you imagine it to be? It could be any number of things, but nothing clearly defined. I've asked thousands of people what they think this is, and responses can be anything from a "cigarette lighter" to a "block falling off some other blocks." In terms of differentiation, we might think of it as a baby's babbling, where there are no recognizable words.

2: A little more differentiation

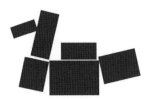

Figure 8.3
A little more differentiation, a few more parts.

In Figure 8.3, you see a bit more differentiation, expressed as the six blocky shapes. What do you suppose it could be? A big mess? Google Earth unfocused? Children's toy blocks scattered on the floor? In terms of differentiation, you might think of it as the baby saying *"gaga,"* which you have learned means "water."

3: Lots more differentiation

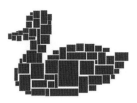

Figure 8.4
Lots more differentiation, many more parts.

As you look at Figure 8.4, it takes little effort to see that this is the form of a duck, though not fully formed. You might think of it as the equivalent amount of differentiation that a baby has for saying "wawa," which most of us would understand to mean "water."

4: Full integration of the duck

Figure 8.5
Integration of the parts into a duck.

Finally, in Figure 8.5, you see a high degree of differentiation, with millions of new connections in the brain fully integrated to create a clear illustration of the duck. This could represent the amount of differentiation and integration the child has learned to clearly say the word "water."

Taking advantage of the brain's remarkable abilities to change for the better

In order to facilitate powerful learning, growth, and transformation in the child, we need to communicate with the brain in its own *language*: movement. We also need to follow the "brain's rules," that is, the way this information system operates. The *Nine Essentials* are principles, conditions, and ways of being and doing. They provide novel ways of interacting with the child, dramatically enhancing their brain's ability to perceive differences, ushering in learning and transformation that may seem miraculous. The *Essentials* are fully supported by current brain research. As Dr Michael Merzenich, pioneer in the field of brain plasticity, wrote in the Foreword to *Kids Beyond Limits*:

> *Scientists have defined the 'rules' governing brain plasticity. We now know how to drive brains to change for the better... My friend Anat Baniel, working in parallel along a completely different path, has defined almost exactly the same rules (The Nine Essentials) in practical human terms.*
>
> Baniel 2012

The *Nine Essentials*

Movement with attention

Movement is the language of the brain. The brain grows, forms, and is organized through movement. Automatic, repetitive movement grooves in already existing patterns. When the child pays attention to what he feels as he moves, his brain immediately starts building millions of new connections that usher in learning and transformation (Nudo et al. 1996). You can use any movement the child is doing, or that you are doing with the child; but direct his attention *to what he feels* as he moves.

Slow

Fast, we can only do what we already know. That is how the brain works. *To learn and master new skills and overcome limitations, the first thing to do is to slow way down.* Slow helps the brain notice differences and gets the child's attention. Slow helps the child's brain get out of its rigidity and compulsivity. You can find multiple opportunities to slow yourself and your child down. Try it and experience how such a seemingly simple shift can make a huge difference.

Variation

Variation – doing different things in different ways – is at the heart of learning (Black et al. 1990, Schilling et al. 2003, Wymbs et al. 2016). It is, in fact, a necessity for learning. Variation generates differences to be perceived, providing the brain with new information. We see enormous variation in the way typical children act. We can call it play, or mistakes, or exploration. By contrast, children with cerebral palsy have little variation in their movements, and children with autism spectrum disorder tend to be rigid, with a limited repertoire of repetitive behaviors depriving their brain of variations with which to learn. When children have difficulty doing or understanding something, rather than asking them to do it the *right* way, *playfully* help them do it in many different "wrong" ways. Then move on to something else with the same intentional, playful approach and witness the brilliance of their brain emerging.

Subtlety

A powerful way to enhance the ability of a child's brain to perceive differences is to reduce the amount of force and intensity in the way you move, talk to, or touch her. *The less the force or intensity, the more the brain can notice changes and perceive differences, empowering it to organize successful action.* This is how I moved Max, Melinda, and Lizzi during their sessions. We often are told, "No pain, no gain." We tend to try harder, to force, to insist on many repetitions in an attempt to achieve outcome. Unfortunately, this makes it more difficult for the brain to perceive differences and for the child to learn and heal.

Enthusiasm

Enthusiasm is self-generated. It is a skill you can develop in yourself, as a parent, teacher, or therapist to help the child's brain learn. Enthusiasm is not clapping your hands, becoming loud and cheering the child on because they did something you wanted. *Enthusiasm is an internal, quiet, and intentional process of amplification* during which you choose to feel delighted about seemingly small or larger changes in the child. The child *feels* your enthusiasm without your saying anything, thus amplifying and helping to "groove in" changes in their brain.

Flexible goals

The pressure to have a child progress according to the expected developmental milestones is enormous. When children aren't performing in accordance with what is expected, often the focus is on trying to get them to do what they *should be able to do, but can't*. When we do this, however, we actually groove in the current limitations in the child, rather than creating new possibilities. I tell parents to stop trying to have the child do what they are unable to do at present: "If he could,

he would; if she could, she would." Instead, start where the child is. Find something, anything, that the child can already do and is interested in and create a learning process around that. You can think about it as *differentiating around the edges of what the child is currently able to do*, thus creating new neural networks from which skills will develop and improve. Flexible goals will also reduce your anxiety, as well as increasing creativity, resulting in greater success, vitality, and joy for all concerned.

The learning switch

The brain is either in a learning mode, when the learning switch is on – or it's not. Stress, fear, multiple repetitions, fatigue, and hunger turn the learning switch off. You know that the switch is on when the child pays attention and becomes interested. *Just a few seconds of clear perception of differences can lead to significant changes.* Whenever you notice that the switch is off, see if using the *Essentials* turns it on. If not, take a break, back off, and come back to it later. Remember Max? When I asked Max whether he wanted to throw the left or right shoe out of the window, it was a surprise, very different from the usual "Don't do that!" warning he heard regularly. With my question about which shoe he wanted to throw, Max's learning switch flipped to on!

Imagination and dreams

Einstein said: "Imagination is everything. It is the preview to life's coming attractions." Imagination requires higher levels of use of the brain and can have just as great or greater an impact on learning as the "real thing." Through imagination the brain grows new neural connections (differentiation) and figures out new possibilities before actually having to perform. When children are very young,

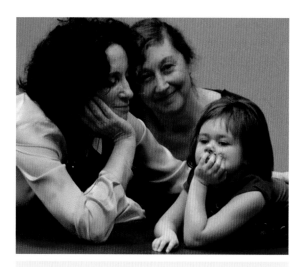

Figure 8.6
Anat Baniel working with a child.

Courtesy of Anat Baniel

the onus for imagining and being creative is on the parent or therapist. Whenever you replace repetitive practices with imagination, you open a door to new possibilities; repetitive actions only groove in existing patterns more deeply. With older children, engage them in imaginative interaction and play. If a child is limited in their ability to imagine, introduce it gradually in small chunks.

Awareness

Awareness is the glue of learning; it is the highest level of functioning of our brain. Awareness is also an action: a thing we do. I coined the word *awaring* – the action of generating awareness. This is the opposite of automaticity and compulsion. Awaring is the ability to be your own observer. For example, it is knowing that you are moving your arm, or raising your voice, and thus having a choice in what you do. Typical children are aware from a very early age, long before they can talk. To help build awareness, try narrating what the child is doing; for example: "You are jumping. You are turning around. You are

crying." Join the child by doing what they are doing, or by asking them whether they want you to join in doing what they are doing. You may also try this: if the child is very loud, ask him to be louder, then even louder, and only then less loud. Remember perception of differences is the source of learning.

All of the *Nine Essentials* are learnable. Practice one at a time, for one week, starting with the first. Look for ways to implement it anywhere you can with yourself and with the child. At the end of the week, proceed to the next Essential and practice that one for a week, while continuing to use the previous ones with which you have already experimented.

Each of the *Nine Essentials* can be applied at home, in the classroom, and during therapy. They are counterintuitive. They represent the shift from a mechanical model to an informational model and from trying to *fix* a child to *connecting with* a child. Give them a try and be pleasantly surprised.

The Anat Baniel Method NeuroMovement practitioner, when working with a child, first of all knows that he or she cannot fix the child. The child is not a machine. Rather, they connect with the child through movement and the *Essentials*, in ways that will help the child's brain do its job better. They always start where the child is, helping to drive differentiation and leading to remarkable, spontaneous "jumps" in skills and development.

References and notes

Baniel, A. 2012. *Kids Beyond Limits*. TarcherPerigee, New York, NY.

Black, J.E., Isaacs, K.R., Anderson, B.J., Alcantara, A.A., Greenough, W.T. 1990. Learning causes synaptogenesis, whereas motor activity causes angiogenesis, in cerebellar cortex of adult rats. *Proceedings of the National Academy of Sciences* 87:5568–5572.

McEwan, M.H., Dihoff, R.E., Brosvic, G.M. 1991. Early Infant crawling experience is reflected in later motor skill development. *Perceptual and Motor Skills* 72:75–79.

(Studies show children who were categorised as early walkers, or those who have crawled for a comparatively short time, demonstrated lower performance scores on preschool assessment tests. This supports the importance of allowing time for the development of sensory and motor systems of the body and general motor skill development.)

Mizrahi, A. 2007. Dendritic development and plasticity of adult-born neurons in the mouse olfactory bulb. *Nature Neuroscience* 10(4):444–452.

(Scientists are able to measure and track the process of differentiation as it is taking place in the brain.)

Nudo, R.J., Milliken, G.W., Jenkins, W.M., Merzenich, M.M. 1996. Use-dependent alterations of movement representations in primary motor cortex of adult squirrel monkeys. *Journal of Neuroscience* 16:785–807.

Prasad, K.N. 1980. *Regulation of differentiation in mammalian nerve cells.* Plenum, NY.

(Differentiation is the capacity of the brain to use information that it acquires through perceiving differences to create new connections between different brain cells. Differentiation is a fundamental process underlying all forms of life.)

Schilling, M.A., Vidal, P., Ployhart, R.E., Marangoni, A. 2003. Learning by doing something else: variation, relatedness, and the learning curve. *Management Science* 49(1):39–56.

Wallace, J.L., Wienisch, M., Murthy, V.N. 2017. Development and refinement of functional properties of adult-born neurons. *Neuron* 96(4):883–896.

(While little is known about the functional development of individual neurons in vivo, recent research supports rapid integration of adult-born neurons into existing circuits, followed by experience-dependent refinement of their functional connectivity.)

Wymbs, N.F., Bastian, A.J., Celnik, P.A. 2016. Motor skills are strengthened through reconsolidation. *Current Biology* 26(3):338–343.

Other resources

(For more information about the *Nine Essentials* and Anat Baniel Method NeuroMovement.)

Baniel, A. 2012. *Kids Beyond Limits.* TarcherPerigee, New York.

Baniel, A. 2016. *Move Into Life: NeuroMovement for Lifelong Vitality,* 2nd edn CreateSpace Independent Publishing Platform, Scotts Valley, CA.

To watch portions of lessons as examples of implementation of the *Nine Essentials*, go to https://www.youtube.com/user/abmethod and watch:

Treatment for Autism in Children – Anat Baniel Method NeuroMovement: holistic autism treatment (Jonathan)

Brachial Plexus Treatment & Anat Baniel Method NeuroMovement: Working with Devorah https://www.youtube.com/watch?v=LPP_77rl-Qc

Anat Baniel Method Foundation: Amy shares the story of her son Cypress https://www.youtube.com/watch?v=8-M-FFxhb0Q

A *NeuroMovement* Video Lesson taught by Anat Baniel

Integrating the Feldenkrais Method® into Scholastic Learning

In 2014, we initiated an innovative project in Israel aiming to change the method of learning in schools. To do this, we introduced movement lessons and ideas from the Feldenkrais Method into weekly classes of mathematics, English, and other topics. Our intention was to realize Moshe Feldenkrais' original vision of integrating the characteristics of organic learning with scholastic learning. The teachers in the project have taught in over 50 classrooms in ten schools around Israel. Here we outline the underlying ideas, principles, and current results of this ongoing project.

Organic learning

What is high-quality learning? We would all like to be able to learn anything we want, with the same depth, soundness and dexterity as we learned, for example, how to walk or speak our mother tongue. Learning is of high quality if the acquired knowledge is available for use in contexts far from those in which the subject was learned, and that this remains true for a long time; if the learner, in some sense, "owns" what was learned and it becomes an "organic" part of them.

Dr Feldenkrais believed that infants and babies learn in the most complete and effective way by what he called *organic learning*. He explained that "organic learning begins in the womb and continues during the whole of the individual's period of physical growth… other forms of learning directed by teachers take place in schools, universities, and colleges…" (Feldenkrais 1981, p. 29). He observed babies, children, and adults (including his own growth) on his journey to discover and define the characteristics of organic learning, and to create a practical method using them.

Perhaps the most important aspect of organic learning in babies is that it is *self-guided*, without judgmental evaluation from the outside. Feldenkrais said, "The organic learning is slow, and unconcerned with any judgment as to the achievement of good or bad results. It has no obvious purpose or goal. It is guided only by the sensation of satisfaction" (Feldenkrais 1981, p. 30). It is the search for a more pleasant and comfortable state of being that guides the learner. The learning happens with ease, and is accompanied with playfulness, attentiveness, and curiosity.

Importantly, high-quality results are derived not by repeating the same action with the hope of achieving perfection but by trying it out in different contexts and variations, integrating it with what the learner already knows. "Each attempt feels less awkward, as the result of avoiding a former minor error which felt unpleasant or difficult" (Feldenkrais 1981, p. 31). Perfection is not a goal; the learning inherently consists of approximations. Moreover, we never know in advance what it is that will be learned. The *field of approximations* is a platform for future actions to be learned. For example, a baby lying on his back starts to roll; following his eyes, he might turn to his side and stay there, exploring possible movements, looking around, reaching for a toy. In the future this will lead him to other actions, like rolling onto his belly, but for now, what the baby does is not perceived by him as an approximation, nor as a failure to do something else; it is experienced as a full action. No external guidance is needed for this personal and intricate learning process.

Scholastic learning in schools

Traditional approaches to teaching, such as the ones practiced in most schools today, evoke learning processes that are quite different from those of a baby. Perhaps the main difference is that self-guidance is replaced by outside guidance, and dependence on the evaluation by teachers. "The students know *what* they learn and when they have achieved the learning to the teacher's satisfaction. Their training is strewn with exercises designed to reach the desired goal to the teacher's satisfaction" (Feldenkrais 1981, p. 31). It is the teacher, rather than the learner, who *leads* the process of learning.

Scholastic learning is a great achievement of humanity. Over tens of thousands of years, humanity has collected huge amounts of knowledge, from logical thinking and arithmetic to craftsmanship and the arts. Ways were invented to transmit this precious knowledge from generation to generation, mainly by having the learner be guided by someone who had previously acquired the knowledge and who could offer shortcuts. However, mankind's main evolutionary advantage is our way of wiring-in our own nervous system, based on self-experience. Slowness and retardation of development are typical characteristics of such a learning process. The human baby begins to walk only about one year after birth, whereas a fawn begins to walk when it is just a few hours old. "Human development is so strongly retarded that even mature adults retain sufficient flexibility for our adaptive status as a learning animal" (Gould 1977, p. 401).

There is an apparent trade-off. Despite the great advantages of scholastic learning, there are pitfalls in the way it is practiced currently in many schools. For many pupils, learning is of poor quality; they are uninterested or not engaged. Many say they feel stupid or that they lack talent in certain topics; and many carry within them, sometimes for years, negative feelings and beliefs about their capabilities, or about academic learning in general.

The starting points for our project were the following questions:

- Is it possible to bring (some of) the characteristics of organic learning into scholastic learning in schools so as to improve the quality of learning as well as the joy and engagement of both pupils and teachers?

- Moreover, can this be done without significantly compromising the curriculum?

- And if so, how can this be implemented methodologically?

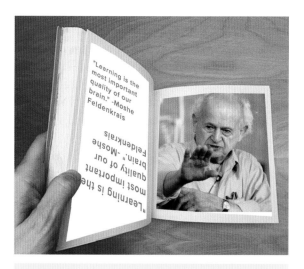

Figure 9.1

"Learning is the most important quality of our brain." Moshe Feldenkrais, Amherst, 1980–81.

Courtesy of Tiffany Sankary

The Feldenkrais Method: a methodological road toward organic learning

Feldenkrais' *Awareness Through Movement* (ATM) lessons offer a methodological way to lead people, even if no longer infants, into a state of organic learning. Each lesson consists of a series of movement instructions, accompanied by directives to sense, listen, and become aware of the way different parts of the body participate in the action, as well as of the interactions with the environment. Typically, after a few movements, there is a resting period which enables an integration of "the new to the old." Thoughts, feelings, emotions, and actions intertwine within the learning process. Gradually, the student's movement ability improves. Importantly, the underlying ability of the student to learn gradually improves, too. Students become more aware of their inner state of being and learn how to create the conditions *they* need in order to attain high-quality learning, which resembles organic learning.

The following ATM lesson was taught for kids aged 5–8 years old. The children were sitting at their desks with paper and pencil and given the following instructions:

1 Draw circles on your paper. Big and small circles. Then put the paper and pencil aside and rest a moment, sitting.

2 Draw circles on the table with one finger. Stop, and draw a circle in the opposite direction.

3 Choose a finger of the other hand and draw small circles and big circles. Now in the opposite direction. Which direction do you like more?

4 Return to the first hand and choose another finger. Draw circles with this finger. Small and big. Now make tiny circles. Change the direction.

5 Now, a surprise. Bring your nose close to the table and draw circles with your nose; you don't have to touch the table. Change the direction. Listen to your neck; is there any movement there? Do you feel your back moving?

6 – 8 Children are given the same instructions, but now with their ears, chin, and elbows.

9 Now take another piece of paper and with a pencil draw circles again.

With many children, the circles drawn at the end of the lesson were more circular. The movement became smoother, with more body parts cooperating harmoniously. *We did not ask the children to make the circles rounder.* Dexterity emerged from doing the action with non-habitual variations, with ease and playfulness; each variation was an engaging challenge, calling for a new non-habitual orchestration of body parts and perception of the action.

Organic learning in schools

In the classes participating in the project, ATM lessons are given weekly and involve both a Feldenkrais teacher and a school teacher. The teachers and pupils do an ATM, then proceed to the subject's lesson, already enhanced with the awareness, attentiveness, and other qualities of organic learning acquired and improved by the ATM lesson.

The idea is that qualities of organic learning can be transferred this way into scholastic learning. Feldenkrais wrote about the possibility of this transfer: "Learning to think in patterns of relationships, in sensations divorced from the fixity of words, allows us to find hidden resources and the ability to make new patterns, to carry over patterns of relationships from one discipline to another" (Feldenkrais 1981, p. 34).

Movement plays a unique role in this possible transfer because of its primary role in arranging the different components of human experience since birth. According to Feldenkrais, ATM constitutes a *meeting point* for our ways of learning in all areas.

The pairs of co-teachers in the project meet weekly to prepare for their joint classes by teaching each other their intended lessons. The role of the Feldenkrais teachers is crucial in these preparatory meetings, since they are familiar with the state of organic learning and can help to create it within the settings by asking simple questions and bringing more awareness into the situation. The co-teachers can then carry over various aspects of this experience of organic learning of the subject matter into the classroom. This preparation also makes them more aware of the students' state during the learning process.

The processes in the classroom

As the year progresses, a common language of attention and awareness begins to develop. The school-teachers become more aware of where the students are in the learning process and of what they *can do easily* rather than what they cannot do; they learn to see what the students *actually do and understand* rather than what they are supposed to do.

An important aspect is the attitude to the state of not-knowing and to mistakes. Moishik Lerner, the third partner in leading this project, who taught mathematics for three years with a Feldenkrais co-teacher, says:

In the Feldenkrais Method, learners are guided to observe and become intimately familiar with their movements. There's no possibility for a mistake in this investigation – it is his or her body, what is comfortable for him or her, and there is no right or wrong. At first, we thought that this

comfort with not-knowing would 'trickle down,' nonverbally, from the movement lesson to the mathematics lesson. We came to realize, however, that we should give the space of error a spoken presence, to instill confidence in the students learning math to set out, observe, and wander without worrying about not knowing which direction to take. And the first thing was to give ourselves – the teachers – the mathematical 'wandering space'; to allow ourselves to be in this state of not-knowing.

As the teachers participate in the ATMs, they become students themselves. In doing so, they too assume the freedom to become learners in the arithmetic, science, or English classes that they teach; and the students also see them as learners. This legitimacy of the state of not-knowing is a source of relief for both the students and the teachers. In particular, students can then ask questions more freely, based on their feelings and associations, which help connect the material to what truly interests *them*.

The ability to be comfortable in the state of not-knowing and making mistakes is closely related to the ability to listen to the different ways others are thinking, without judgment. Classes in the project involve many discussions in small groups, in which the pupils explain what they understood, and discuss difficult points. They learn to listen to each other with more interest and ask detailed questions about how their friends understand things. One exercise we use is to instruct the pupils to explain to a partner in detail how they solved a simple exercise, like 137 minus 52. The listener has to try to understand the way his or her partner was thinking, without trying to correct them.

All this creates a growing freedom, for both students and teachers in the classroom, to express their abilities and feelings. Notera Michaeli, a teacher of mathematics in our project, said:

After the ATM with the children I feel more at ease... We work now, often, in small groups, which I did before only seldomly because it requires high concentration from the pupils. I was surprised by how quiet and calm they are... I became much more creative during the lesson. I discovered that I now feel freer to change things, also because of the state of the pupils.

One may ask whether all of this does not slow the learning too much, or make it less effective; but in fact all the classes in our project in which pupils and teachers successfully engaged in the Feldenkrais lessons learned *more* than the usual curriculum, and the teachers thought that the quality of the learning was higher.

Where we go next

We have seen a far-reaching impact on students and teachers alike, at both the sensory and experiential levels, as well as in terms of their achievements. This is exciting and encouraging. Clearly, the methods we have developed for the transfer of learning skills from the movement to scholastic learning are still rudimentary, and more is required before this can be used on a large scale. Nevertheless, we believe our results so far give very encouraging indications that the Feldenkrais Method could offer profound improvements in the way learning is accomplished in schools today.

References

Feldenkrais, M. 2019. *The Elusive Obvious.* Reprint. North Atlantic Books/Somatic Resources, San Francisco.

Gould, S.J. 1977. *Ontogeny and Phylogeny.* Harvard University Press, Cambridge, MA.

Other resources

Almagor, E. Learning Through Movement in Class. YouTube video; search for "Almagor Sequence 01" https://www.youtube.com/watch?v=BeIMxK3HwPA&feature=youtu.be [Accessed October 9, 2020]

Almagor, E. Learning Through Movement in Class. YouTube video; search for "Ohad Yad Hamore": https://www.youtube.com/watch?v=fkY1wox9iSs&feature=youtu.be [Accessed October 9, 2020]

Introduction

Movement is not something human beings should take for granted. Unlike other living creatures that are able to stand on their feet and walk immediately after birth, human babies are responsible for learning the skill of movement all by themselves. They do this through a process of trial and error, exploring many options until they finally arrive at movements that serve their needs and satisfy their urges. Beyond accomplishing their aims, human babies' autonomous quests also develop in them a "movement intelligence" that becomes their ever-faithful compass for navigating coordination throughout a future filled with unforeseen events.

Civilized humans, living under the minimal physical demands of modern society, have discontinued this process of trial and error and instead rely on daily routines, which, though they may not be optimally efficient, serve their existence. In time this compromised way of life can lead to serious health complications. In order not to deteriorate, humans need to use their bodies constantly and to their fullest potential. The inescapable law of nature applies: *What you do today becomes easier to do tomorrow; what you don't today becomes more difficult tomorrow.* To maintain adequate function, a person must persist in perfecting their quality of moving, as well as in nurturing their passion to do so. Physical fitness is a dynamic, ongoing process. It is less like stashing your hard-earned cash away in a bank's safe-deposit box and more like having the ability to raise capital whenever needed, coupled with knowing how to invest it wisely and sensibly throughout a lifetime's worth of unpredictable twists, turns, ups and downs.

In offering his solutions for the deteriorating quality of modern man's movement, Moshe Feldenkrais modeled his strategies on the auto-didactic processes that occur naturally in the human baby. He deciphered the ingredients of the formulae for developing functional fitness from the way this happens spontaneously, in nature, and applied these same organic principles of original habit formation to modifying and upgrading a matured human's lifetime accumulation of ingrained, often dysfunctional, habits.

The somatic learning of the subconscious

Feldenkrais' main observation was that the natural development of movement skill during the early stages of life occurs in a totally autonomous, self-directed way – in the primal, preverbal layers of the brain, without relying on any external guidance. Acquisition of movement skill thus results from the dialogue between a specific internal urge (its motivation) and the qualitative sensory feedback that accompanies a child's attempts to satisfy this urge. Children arrive at an acceptable pattern of moving only after a period of trial and error, during which they explore a range of options, comparing and contrasting sensory feedback. In order for a particular pattern of coordination to become consolidated and store itself into functional memory for future use as a dependable habit, children first need to feel and trust that any new pattern adequately serves their intention. This determination is only arrived at after a personally experienced sense of comfort and safety, which confirms that a desirable coordination has indeed been achieved, not just satisfactorily but also satisfyingly. The qualitative "how" is as important as the quantitative "what." This principle, of trusting the individual's auto-selection process, is what sets Feldenkrais' approach apart from other methods of somatic inquiry and fitness development that prescribe a pre-ordained "right" model, which tend to cultivate movement potential through the adoption and incorporation of external principles rather than by encouraging individuals to evolve themselves uniquely, from within, in a more natural, dignified, and significantly less authoritarian way.

The Feldenkrais Method applies a human baby's autonomous learning method to mature adults, including those who suffer from a wide range of functional limitations. Students are guided to intentionally explore numerous, varied movement themes or lessons, and in so doing clarify the full range of their anatomic possibilities. These open exploration – conducted safely and within a student's comfort zone – avoiding the direct pursuit of a "correct" solution. Instead, the intention is to *awaken the organism's innate judgment mechanism*, transcending habitual ways of responding and moving, and leading the student to trust in – and rely upon – their own deeper internal resources.

Distinct from a baby's innate learning process, the adult's relearning process occurs simultaneously at the levels of cognitive awareness and subjective sensation. Only after being guided to explore unused options that loosen rigid patterns of physical behavior – ones the body has been relying upon for years – is an adult's subconscious ready to accept the possibility of organizing itself differently. Refining the management of body movement in this manner reconnects a student with the primal wisdom within that already knows how to seek out behavior best suited for life. It also redirects a maturing human being to the ongoing search for improvement, harkening back to childhood.

Integration – the key to organic reorganization

Feldenkrais used nature's most characteristic organizing principle of organic life: the quality of *integration*. From the perspective of integration, a living body coordinates its actions through a network of interrelationships in which each part both affects and is affected by all the others. With an integrative approach, the ability to change – and restore function in – a specific isolated area relies upon a global reconfiguration that recruits the harmonious support and cooperation from every other part of the body, and presupposes the ability and readiness of these parts to adjust themselves accordingly.

The Bones for Life program
Cultivating bone strength and weight-bearing posture

For many years I was a classical Feldenkrais trainer, conducting professional training worldwide and certifying teachers to spread the Feldenkrais Method. After 30 years of teaching in the top echelon of the Feldenkrais world, my attention was drawn to the medical problem of osteoporosis. In response to the growing incidence of bone deterioration and fractures throughout Western society, I began searching for a movement-based solution to this debilitating dysfunction. In this chapter, we consider *Movement Intelligence* concepts originally developed for the Bones for Life program to cultivate bone strength and functional posture, which also promotes graceful, elegant aging.

In creating the Bones for Life program, my intention was to reconcile two complementary needs: gentleness, for somatic learning on the floor, and pressure, to support real-world standing and walking in verticality.

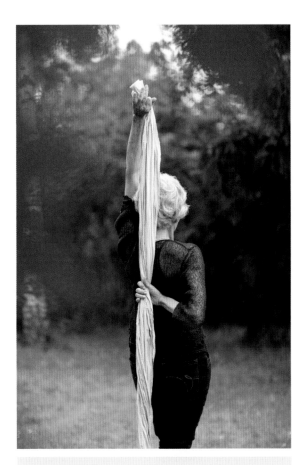

Figure 10.1
The Bones Wrap serves here as an objective visual and tactile guide for upright balance, for toning the extensors of the upper back, and as a cue to engage the "anti-gravity" network of sphincter muscles.

Courtesy of Ruthy Alon

How can out-of-condition people learn to perform dynamic movement?

The most crucial issue addressed in the Bones for Life program is how to guide people whose posture is prone to collapsing at vulnerable joints with their every step; people who have neglected physical fitness for many years and have become used to a compromised way of living in their bodies. How

can they carry out dynamic movement without harming themselves further, without hurting their vulnerable joints, and without causing their deteriorated posture to deteriorate even further?

This is where the unique contributions of the Bones for Life program come to the fore, offering neuromotor strategies that safely secure the body in-action, and presenting learning strategies to awaken from within new choices for reorganizing, restructuring, and redesigning posture. The program offers many simple, focused processes that bypass dysfunction, safely granting students the real-world experience of "antigravity" vertical activity, loaded with power, and carried out in dynamic contexts that support and strengthen the functioning of their bones.

Themes to cultivate bone strength and upright posture

A) Bouncing on the heels – pulsations of pressure build bone

"Vibro-gymnastics" was a technique invented by Russian space engineer Alexander Mikulin to improve circulation. By bouncing on his heels from a height of only one centimeter, he found that the increased pressure into his legs aided circulation; it helped pump blood up through his veins, against gravity, reducing his heart's workload and preventing blood from pooling stagnantly in his feet.

The Bones for Life program uses this very same strategy – rhythmic pulsations, loaded with short bursts of intense pressure – to accomplish three aims: improve circulation, build bone, and optimize posture. "Bouncing on the heels" is our foundational bread-and-butter exercise. We revisit it throughout the program in a range of variations that satisfy the body's need for novelty, as well as its need for repetition in learning. Each new refinement in postural reorganization that the program introduces is affirmed by literally *stamping* it into our consciousness, using the dynamic context of heel bouncing. Our heel bouncing is done in double-pulses – iambic taps that echo the "lub-dub" rhythm of the heartbeat. This familiar pattern is first heard in our mother's womb, which makes it more palatable for our organism to absorb and assimilate.

Heel bouncing strengthens not only our circulation but also the resistance of our bones throughout the entire skeletal system, enabling them to withstand increasingly powerful impacts. Heel bouncing promotes stability in our body by organizing our bones more sensibly – stacked one atop the other, into a better aligned posture; it also generates a joyful feeling and globally refreshes and revitalizes the functions of our entire body.

This activity is easier to perform than either walking or running; almost anyone can bounce on their heels. Even people who have difficulty moving, or who have balance issues and are concerned or even fearful about losing equilibrium and falling, have ready access to a wall or chair to support themselves while they bounce lightly. Bouncing on the heels is the Bones for Life program's essential exercise; it is used with many variations and is regularly assigned as home practice.

B) Postural alignment – prerequisite for safe, dynamic movement

There is no pill for posture; there is no drug that can remedy the way you stand. Your relationship with gravity is your "postural fingerprint," so personal that it presents to the world, beyond all pretense, the characteristic details of your unique way of being in the world. The way your posture is perceived by others stems from the same primordial system that guides survival in the wild – a vital orientation to the environment, a "gut reaction" that rapidly reads a situation and reacts before the slower conscious mind even has time to realize what's going on, let alone respond.

From a physiological standpoint, a streamlined posture is the safest structure with which to produce springy, powerful, bone-building movement. Only when the skeletal frame is well organized is it possible to use movement to vibrate our bones with force strong enough to enhance their resistance to withstand pressure and prevent collapse. Optimal posture cannot be fashioned consciously, by simply repositioning oneself in accord with some external authority. Instead, for it to be adopted and put to use in a meaningful, lasting way, ideal posture needs to be *discovered* – selected unconsciously from within, based on a personally felt relevance to our life, and determined through sensation.

A significant part of the Bones for Life program is devoted to aligning posture in a precise, yet fluidly adaptive way that serves the body in dynamic motion. Posture is not static; it is the result of the sum total of our movement range and quality. When we take the entire body into account, so as to

---

Bouncing on the heels

You might like to hold on to a support during this exercise, to relieve yourself from concern about your balance.

- While standing, lift your heels very slightly from the floor; then drop them back down, with a very light bump.

- Invite your body to remain firm, acting as a single, one-unit block.

- Bounce your heels with double-taps, in a heartbeat rhythm, as you say aloud, "Pum-pum, Pum-pum."

- When you have had enough, stop, stand, and appreciate the difference from when you began. (How is your posture? Your attitude? How long can you remain like this, in comfort, with an attitude of acceptance for this new way of standing?)

secure harmonious interaction among all its components, optimal posture is actually in effect each moment we are in motion. Thus, with ideally well-organized coordination, all our daily activities can become means for strengthening our bones.

Aligning the neck's cervical vertebrae

- While sitting, place one hand behind your neck and explore its shape with your fingers. Locate the deepest point in your cervical curve.

- Place the opening of your other hand at your chin, with your thumb on one cheek, and your index finger on the other.

- With this hand gently guide your chin closer to your throat; to maintain the verticality of your face, you may open your mouth.

- See if you can bring your wrist to your sternum and attach your pinky to your collarbone. Rest your forearm and elbow on your chest.

- With both hands in place, repeat withdrawing your chin several times.

- Feel the change in your neck with the hand behind you. See if you can interpret this as a lengthening of your neck, which is now better aligned and more continuous with your spine.

- Confirm this change by performing an activity in this position:

  - As you get up to stand, maintain a fixed distance between chin and chest; the position of your hands blocks any articulation within your neck.

  - As a result, other larger segments of your spine are recruited for this antigravity task.

  - Still coaxing your chin back with your hand (holding it closer to your chest to straighten your neck while you move) step in place, from one foot to the other. Movement always reinforces the configuration that performs it.

- Finally, take your hands away, and feel how your body chooses to stand. Listen to the statement your posture now makes.

Decompressing the lower back's lumbar vertebrae

- Stand in a "step position" – one foot in front of the other, as if taking a step – and allow your knees to unlock.

- Put the back of the hand on the same side as your back leg at the curve of your lumbar region: the little finger at the sacrum, and the thumb resting just above your waistline. Bend your knees slightly.

- Allow your fingers, attached to the tissues of your lower back, to spread open the spaces between them; they encourage elongation of the lumbar spine, which occurs in response to a change in the position of your pelvis.

- Repeat this several times.

- Each time you straighten your knees, your fingers approach each other; acknowledge your lumbar spine getting shorter. Each time you bend your knees, your fingers separate, dragging along with them the tissues they touch.

- Now keep your knees unlocked all the time. Put your other hand on your belly: your little finger at the bottom of your belly, thumb above your navel.

- Squeeze together the tissues of your belly, the hand on your front bringing the thumb and little finger together while the hand on your back feels the response in your lumbar spine.

Shortening your front leads to the release and lengthening of your back.

- Repeat this several times. Maintain the squeezed position and confirm the elongation of your lumbar spine by stepping in place.

- To further enhance the decompression of your lumbar region, bend both knees with each stepping foot. Do this minimally, in a way that corresponds with your natural way of walking.

- Finally, stand and feel what has changed in your posture. Perhaps you notice that your pelvis hangs lower than usual. Maybe you discover that your knees no longer tend to lock, compulsively, as in the past; they might even be like springs.

- Walk around to experience new sensations in your lower back.

C) Basic patterns of locomotion – Wave and Axis

The Bones for Life program differentiates two modes of mobilization: "Wave" and "Axis." The flexible, undulating Wave mode is used for swimming, crawling, and walking. The Axis mode – which firms up the skeleton into a solid unit – is used for antigravity tasks like fast walking or jumping. Underscoring the distinction between Wave and Axis clarifies our movement management and sharpens our comprehension of these two complementary modes. Wave movement – which allows the spine to smoothly undulate, for flexibility – serves forward propulsion. In contrast, axial movement – which lifts our body weight to outsmart gravity, as in jumping – functions when we are upright, in the vertical plane.

Our joints are designed for flexibility. Each neighboring pair of bones has a unique degree of

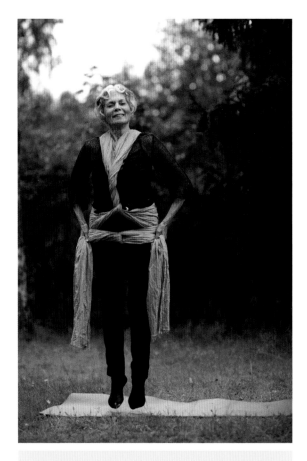

Figure 10.2
Streamlining the body with the Bones Wrap facilitates the difficult earthly physical challenge: jumping. Think *down* to spring up and exhale – Ha!

Courtesy of Ruthy Alon

freedom and opens to an anatomically prescribed distance; in aggregate, they facilitate our total body locomotion. But our joints also play another role. In certain functions they lock – tightening bones together, one to its neighbor, binding them into a single unit – and so they must also be able to *forgo* their ability to articulate. In this opposing function, our joints serve stability, rather than mobility; they fasten our bones to each other and are responsible for aligning our skeleton in a continuously stream-lined, firm, and unbendable axis – a unified struc-ture that can safely bear the increased workload of lifting our entire body weight. This locking phase of our joints positions our bones to their best mechan-ical advantage – where they are able to withstand a high degree of pressure and resist collapse in the gravitational field. Functioning in this stabilized Axis mode trains our bones to fulfill their destiny and form the strong, solid structure that shapes and supports our body architecture from within.

Moving in the Axis mode demands sophisticated neuromuscular control and finely regulated man-agement of power. Though part of the Bones for Life program is devoted to cultivating wave-like proportional flexibility among our joints, it is also essential to learn to configure the spine into a firm, solid axis.

The Axis mode is first learned lying on the floor – in safe "greenhouse" conditions – where one leg or hand pushes a wall gradually and sensitively. It is then possible to feel how the entire body becomes loaded with streaming force – though never to a degree that breathing is disturbed. The body becomes straighter and better aligned as the spinal curves begin to lengthen toward the objective plane of the floor. Another protective set of greenhouse conditions for learning to load the axis with deter-mined force comes from standing near a wall. In addition to being able to lean on it for support in the upright plane, the wall also offers an objective ver-tical model for more optimal alignment. Improved posture is further cultivated by practicing numer-ous processes, all conducted against, and with the support of, a wall.

D) Protecting vulnerable joints – safety first

If the vertebrae of the neck are excessively com-pressed under the weight of the forward head; or some upper back vertebrae are bound together; or a specific vertebra in the lumbar spine is too free and thus hypermobile; or there is a combination of these… what chance does the lower back have *but* to react with an exaggerated friction in the recoil of every walking step, despite one's best efforts to try to avoid any strong impact with the ground?

Similarly, if the hip joint, knee, or ankle is too tight or loose, or causes pain with each step, what

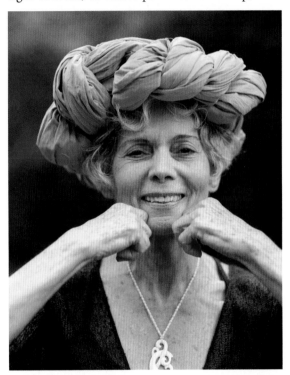

Figure 10.3
A well-aligned spine supports not only the head, but any weight balanced atop – here, a cloth "crown" made from the Bones Wrap. The feather light touch of our hands counters any tendency for cervical instability and collapse by offering direc-tion from the front of our neck that invites it to lengthen in the back.

Courtesy of Ruthy Alon

chance is there that we will find any pleasure in walking?

Before setting out to increase bone strength, by stimulating skeletal resistance to gravity, we need to secure the safety of all our vulnerable joints and involve them in movement as best we can. As its main contribution, the Bones for Life program offers a comprehensive set of unique strategies that address all areas of potential disharmony in order to ensure the safety and efficiency of all parts of the skeletal system. From this perspective it can be seen that, to accomplish its mission of *safely* strengthening bone tissue, this program entails a reorganization that upgrades, repairs, and heals the biomechanics of the entire body.

E) Developing skeletal resilience and resistance to bone fracture

The phenomenon of women who transport heavy loads on their heads has been the subject of numerous studies, some of which have shown that they can carry up to 70 percent of their body mass – with corresponding increases in energy consumption related to the borne weight. More surprisingly, research has also shown the comparative bone fracture rate of these water-carrying women to be only one percent of the fracture rate of women in the West (Aspray et al. 1996) – this despite their average bone density not being any higher than that of their Western counterparts. Such a finding leaves us with a curious puzzle: if it is not the *quantitative* density of bone cells, the mass per cubic centimeter, that is significant in preventing bone breakage, then what might be the *qualitative* factors that grant the water carriers their apparent immunity to skeletal fracture?

Certainly, the women have conditioned themselves to carrying heavy loads through a gradual yet consistent process of presenting their bones with

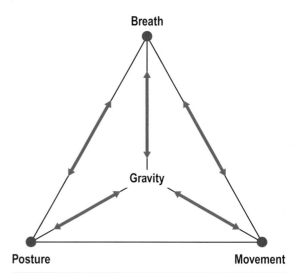

Figure 10.4
Our innate Movement Intelligence artfully negotiates the inviolable framework of interdependent relationships between gravity, posture, movement, and breath, each of which influences the others, strongly to subtly.

Courtesy of Doug Boltson

increasing challenges. But there are additional factors that may be related to the ability of the water carriers' bones to resist fracture – in particular, their style of walking. The rhythmic and graceful pattern of self-mobilization they employ flows in an economic, undulating wave, one that radiates effortlessness as it recurs in regular harmonic cycles. Their smooth, continuous movements attest to the utility of organizing posture in an efficient way, congruently aligned with skeletal design, channeling their mobilizing forces in a functional, streamlined trajectory that is both elegant and simple.

Movement Intelligence

In the entire suite of *Movement Intelligence* programs there are never any intense stretches or acrobatic twists, no goals to pursue and measure, nor prolonged, extreme, sustained positions. Our programs promote function, not achievement. Their aim is to restore the profound underlying biodynamics that constitute evolved patterns of locomotion, offering a pragmatic approach to posture and movement whose purpose is to directly serve everyday living.

When following in nature's footsteps to better mobilize ourselves, we benefit not only from the specifics of a newly acquired configuration but also from the awakening of our inborn talent to create functional harmony – streamlined movement that is applicable to, and enhances, all aspects of our lives. It is our innate ability to globally orchestrate this coordination of many moving parts that we call Movement Intelligence.

Ruthy Alon 1930–2020

Since the writing of this chapter, we have lost Ruthy, one of the most beloved members of the Feldenkrais community. As one of Moshe Feldenkrais' original students, her insight into the work was profound. She continued to learn throughout her life, bringing this work to the public and making it easily accessible for everyone. Ruthy always taught with loving kindness and generosity. Her dedication to Moshe's work, from the early years of her training in Israel to her ongoing work as a trainer and teacher, will continue to influence future generations of learners.

References

Aspray, T.J., Prentice, A., Cole, T.J., Sawo, Y., Reeve, J., Francis, R.M. 1996. Low Bone Mineral Content Is Common but Osteoporotic Fractures Are Rare in Elderly Rural Gambian Women. *Journal of Bone Mineral Research* 11(7):1019–1025.

Other resources

Alon, R. 2018. *Mindful Spontaneity: Lessons in the Feldenkrais Method*. North Atlantic Books, Berkeley, CA.

Freeing the Neck From Behind *Awareness Through Movement* Video Lesson taught by Ruthy Alon
Courtesy of Feldenkrais Access,
https://www.feldenkraisaccess.com/

Chrish's interview with Linda

CHRISH: *Linda, tell us how you came to the Feldenkrais Method?*

LINDA: I first experienced the Feldenkrais Method at the Esalen Institute in 1973 during a workshop taught by Ilana Rubenfeld. One evening, she led us through a Feldenkrais *Awareness Through Movement* (ATM) lesson, and when I stood up after that one-hour lesson, I could move my pelvis like never before! The change in my flexibility was miraculous. I was a professional horse-riding instructor and before I integrated Feldenkrais into my riding, I sat on the horse in a fixed position. That one ATM was life-changing, and that night I danced to rock 'n' roll music like I had never dreamed of dancing before. I can still feel it 46 years later.

What led you to enroll in the Feldenkrais Professional Training Program in San Francisco in 1975?

That one ATM lesson at Esalen played a significant role in my decision to enroll in the Feldenkrais training. But it was actually Roger Russell (a Feldenkrais Trainer currently based in Germany), my partner at that time, who was responsible for my decision to sign up for the training.

It was an unlikely move on my part, as I came from the world of horses, and I enrolled thinking I could use the Feldenkrais Method to enhance the balance and athletic ability of my riding students.

In 1974 I had shut down my international residential school for riding instructors in California and, at age 35, went on "walkabout" to Europe, hoping to discover my soul's purpose on the planet.

In Germany, however, I was pulled back into the horse world by an invitation to direct a new school to teach the style of balanced seat riding that was the hallmark of my California training center.

Roger, inspired by the ATM lesson at Esalen, enrolled in the four-year San Francisco Feldenkrais training, intending to introduce the Feldenkrais Method to German riders in the new school I was to head.

When I read the brochure describing the course at the Humanistic Psychology Institute in San Francisco, I was struck by an intuitive "knowing" that I must also enroll.

I had no inkling that I would develop a new form of training for horses. Nor could I imagine that in the ensuing 45 years my work would spread around the world.

What was the impetus that started you on this different path for training horses?

On the second day of the Feldenkrais training in San Francisco, I remember lying on the floor with my 62 classmates, being led by Moshe through an ATM lesson. He made a statement that made me prick up my ears: "A human's potential for learning can be enhanced, and learning time shortened dramatically, with gentle, non-habitual movements that activate new neural pathways to the brain, thereby developing new brain cells and increasing one's capacity for learning." Wow! When I heard this statement, my first thought was, "What movements could I do with a horse that would be 'non-habitual' and increase a horse's willingness and capacity for learning?"

I love recalling this, because it was a major milestone moment in my life. In 1965, my first husband, Wentworth Tellington, and I published a ground-breaking book entitled *Physical Therapy for the Athletic Horse*, a first in the world of horse-training. It was very effective for physical recovery, but it never crossed my mind that it would be possible to influence the personality, behavior, and attitude of a horse by working on its body until that auspicious day in July 1975 in San Francisco with Moshe.

After class on the second day of the training, Roger and I drove an hour south to Woodside to explore the possibility of applying non-habitual movements on a horse, with the goal of enhancing a horse's ability to learn and affect its personality. I chose a 16-year-old mare who was hard to catch in the pasture and didn't trust people. So, I thought, "Where should I begin?" I had experienced surprising success working on the ears of horses for colic, but never considered working on a horse's ears with the idea of establishing trust.

I remember looking at that horse and thinking, "What can I do with the ears that would develop her ability to trust?" I was looking for ways to move her body that could activate new neural pathways in order to enhance her capacity for learning. As I was listening to Moshe's voice in my head, I began by moving the ears in various directions, gently. Then I directed my attention to her legs, and though we'd been doing physical therapy movements with the legs for years, I now moved them with the Feldenkrais principle of awareness. Next came the tail, and lastly the head and neck. People watching thought I had hypnotized the horse, as she was so focused and quiet.

The next day the owner called me and said "Linda, I don't know what you did to my horse.

When I went to catch her after you left, for the first time ever she was waiting at the gate. Instead of diving for the hay in the corner of the stall, she lowered her head toward me, as though she was saying, 'Touch my ears'."

She had learned to trust in less than an hour. And I thought, "That's interesting: new learning, totally new learning."

That summer after our Feldenkrais classes, I searched for horses with a variety of behavior issues. One of the huge breakthroughs came with a horse belonging to one of the top polo players in California. His mare would not step over a pole on the ground or a line drawn in the sand, so of course she was an interesting challenge for me.

One afternoon I was in the riding arena working with this horse and Roger was standing at her head. There was a jump pole on the ground in front of her that she had refused to step over earlier. Her head was up with a stiff neck and braced body. I intuitively went to her tail and began moving it from the root, making a connection through the spine to her head. Suddenly she dropped her head and stepped over the pole. Wow! That was the beginning of what years later I recognized as the shift from the sympathetic (fight/flight/freeze) state to the parasympathetic (rest and digest), also a state of trust. All I had done was move her tail in a non-habitual way – and her behavior changed.

Roger and I explored many possibilities for moving horses using non-habitual movements that summer. Back in Germany, we continued to develop new concepts for training the horses who came to my workshops. Roger was also totally dedicated to practicing the ATMs himself and kept me inspired.

How were you personally impacted by your studies with Moshe?

During the summers in San Francisco I watched Moshe give *Functional Integration* lessons after class to people who came to him from all over the world. I had the good fortune to receive at least 10 lessons from him myself. It was a hundred bucks a pop for 20 minutes, and in those days that was a lot of money, but worth every penny. I was grateful that he would take me because he wouldn't work with you just for the money. Perhaps he chose me because he knew I was exploring this non-habitual learning concept with horses.

There were many poignant moments in the training. During the first summer I fell asleep a lot, and Moshe said, "It doesn't matter, you'll integrate just as much in your sleep." I was deeply touched that he never judged us for falling asleep.

An unforgettable highlight of the four-year training was the day Moshe lay on the Feldenkrais table and took us through a riveting process, describing how he had come to a state of self-awareness; listening to his body – sensing and feeling as he demonstrated the movements

that had led to the recovery from his knee injury. I can still picture 62 of my classmates sitting on the floor around him, mesmerized. You could have heard a pin drop!

At the end of our first summer of training, Moshe gave us a list of books to read. One of them was *Man on his Nature,* by Nobel prize recipient Sir Charles Sherrington. His concept of cellular intelligence gifted me with the inspiration which is at the heart of the Tellington Basic TTouch Circle. In the second chapter, "Body Wisdom," his premise is, "Every cell in the body knows its function in the body." I was reading this chapter in a Mövenpick restaurant in Stuttgart, Germany, on a rainy winter day. The impact of that statement was overpowering. In that moment I recalled watching a fascinating lesson the previous summer when Moshe worked with a 28-year-old woman suffering from a stroke. The change after a 30-minute session was awe-inspiring.

I put the book down and sat back, holding my hand up and looking at the tips of my fingers. I remember thinking, "Wow! When I don't know yet how to do this amazing Feldenkrais work, all I have to do is talk to my cells when touching

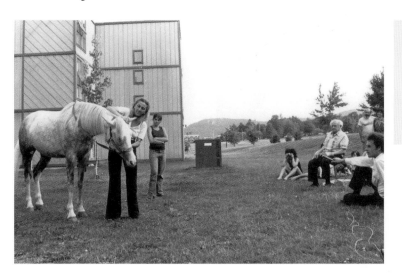

Figure 11.1
Linda Tellington-Jones working with a horse during the Amherst training, Moshe Feldenkrais observing.

Courtesy of Linda Tellington-Jones

another being and remind the cells of their potential for ideal function."

The role of cellular intelligence is at the heart of the Tellington TTouch work. When I put my hands on a person or an animal, I choose to see only their potential for ideal function at the cellular level.

Fascinating! So how did TTouch come about?

Tellington TTouch was "officially" birthed on a warm July day in 1983 at the Delaware Equine Veterinary Clinic. I was asked to work on a reactive horse belonging to one of the veterinarians. This mare objected to grooming or saddling by pinning her ears and threatening to kick. I was asked if I could help her using the Feldenkrais Method. When I placed my hands on her back and began with gentle movements of *Functional Integration*, the mare became uncharacteristically quiet and accepting. Her owner, Wendy, was amazed and asked, "What are you doing to affect my mare in this way? Are you using energy, or what is your secret?"

Without thinking I responded with, "Place your hand lightly on her shoulder and move the skin in a circle."

Moving the skin in a circle was not related to the Feldenkrais Method, but I had learned to trust my intuition, so I watched as Wendy followed my minimal instructions. To my surprise, the mare became as accepting of the light circles as she had been for my Feldenkrais movements.

I had been teaching non-habitual movements that are the mark of the Feldenkrais Method with great success, but in that prophetic moment, when I saw the powerful effects of the circular movements of the skin, I had the intuitive knowing that this was to be my path forward.

From that day on I began experimenting with a variety of circular movements. What has emerged over almost four decades is the Tellington Method, comprised of four components: the TTouch body work with 20-plus hand positions combined with varying tempos and pressures that anyone can learn; ground exercises called the Playground for Higher Learning to enhance focus and balance

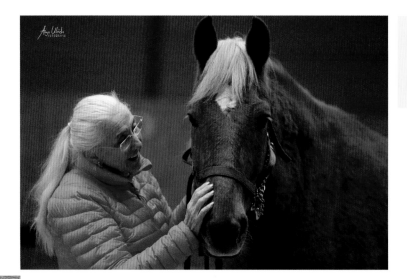

Figure 11.2
Linda Tellington-Jones with one of her beloved horses.

Courtesy of Linda Tellington-Jones

for horses and dogs; specialized equipment; and the TTouch philosophy: "Change the posture and you can change the behavior of your horse or dog," and "You must change your mind in order to change the behavior, performance, relationship or well-being of your animals or yourself."

The Tellington TTouch Method crosses the species barrier and has spread around the globe, applicable for humans as well as all animals. I remember Moshe saying, "Don't just do my work, develop your own fingerprints." I believe he would be proud of his influence on the Tellington Method. Thank you, Moshe, for your gifts to the world.

Other resources

Bodin, L., Bodin Lamboy, N., Graciet, J. 2016. *The Book of Ho'oponopono: The Hawaiian practice of forgiveness and healing.* Destiny Books, Rochester, VT.

Braden, G. 2006. *Secrets of the Lost Mode of Prayer: The hidden power of beauty, wisdom, and hurt.* Hay House, Carlsbad, CA.

Byron, K., Mitchell, S. 2003. *Loving What Is: Four questions that can change your life.* Three Rivers Press, New York.

Jampolsky, G.G. 2010. *Love Is Letting Go of Fear*, 3rd edn. Celestial Arts, Toronto.

Miller, R.L. 2020. *Uncommon Prayer*, 3rd edn. Portal Center Press, Waldport, OR.

O'Bryan, T. 2018. *You Can Fix Your Brain: Just 1 hour a week to the best memory, productivity, and sleep you've ever had.* Rodale Books, Emmaus, PA.

Tellington-Jones, L. 2012 *Getting in TTouch with Your Dog: A gentle approach to influencing behavior, health and performance*, 2nd edn. Trafalgar Square Books, North Pomfret, VT.

Tellington-Jones, L., Pretty, M. 2019. *Training and Retraining Horses the Tellington Way: Starting Right or Starting Over with Enlightened Methods and Hands-On Techniques.* Trafalgar Square Books, North Pomfret, VT.

Wendler, M.C, Tellington-Jones, L. 2008. *TTouch for Healthcare: The healthcare professional's guide to Tellington TTouch®.* Tellington TTouch Training, Santa Fe, NM.

Heart Hug *TTouch* Video Lesson and Talk by Linda Tellington-Jones

Anxiety, stress, trauma, worry, and acute or chronic physical pain are hallmarks of our modern human condition. Having ample energy to enjoy life, relationships, families, friends, and hobbies along with accomplishing daily goals is something we all desire. We try to seek relief through self-help books, medication, therapy, vacations, burnout recovery clinics, and technological distractions. These solutions can be effective at times; we needn't eliminate them. However, there is a missing ingredient that would potentiate all of the above: *movement*. But not just any movement: a specifically designed method to move yourself in new directions of thinking, sensing, and feeling, toward action that will help control or eliminate habits that are not beneficial.

Our habits are built upon past events which caused us to develop faulty thinking and emotional reactions that may have outgrown their usefulness or become emotionally and physically painful in themselves. In fact, regardless of whether the pain we are experiencing is emotional or physical, the same area of the brain reacts: the anterior cingulate cortex, which is part of the limbic system. This part of the brain is interconnected with the amygdala and the hypothalamus and is thought to be involved with a number of functions related to assigning meaning to emotions and internal and external stimuli, as well as the selection and initiation of motor movements. Someone's unkind words make us feel like we've been punched in the gut. More pleasantly, falling in love gives us butterflies in our tummies. Emotions represent excitation in the nervous system; like waves, they vary in strength – they come and go. Sensations, emotions, and movement are intertwined (Siegel 2015). These elements are woven into the tapestry of our lives. Redesigning that tapestry, however, can be liberating.

Case Study: Sally changes her self-image

Here is a glimpse of the Feldenkrais Method of somatic education with Sally, a 42-year-old married woman with two young children. A busy mom, she also enjoys part-time work in a boutique. At our first session, she said: "My husband is supportive, but he spends long hours at his law practice. I have plenty of women friends, and I'm mostly happy."

"What would you like to learn, Sally?" My question prompted participating in a *learning* relationship rather than a therapeutic treatment model, wherein she would expect me to treat her problems.

She looked at me quizzically and replied: "I want to feel my body more. I think I am afraid to. Sometimes I feel anxious and kind of numb – separated from my body. Can I learn to feel more comfortable in my own skin? Using your word, can I "*learn*" to have sexual desire for my husband?" She added, laughing, "It would make us both happier. I feel physically tired and especially tense in my hips, shoulders and neck; maybe this interferes with our sex life."

I repeated her request, to let her know I understood. "Yes, you can learn to feel more fully, sense yourself comfortably and cultivate sexual desire for your husband. During your lesson, you will start to understand how this can occur."

I asked Sally to share some important moments in her life. "Falling in love with my husband, having babies, traveling in Europe before meeting my husband. On the downside, my stepfather raped me when I was sixteen. When I told my mother, she kicked him out of the house. We never reported him – I regret that, but we were scared. I don't know if I am completely over that experience, but I rarely think of it. I did some counseling at the time."

Many people who have experienced sexual trauma do not realize the impact these traumas may have on current behaviors.

While Sally spoke, I listened attentively, summarized and reflected what she shared. Her breathing deepened and she settled into her chair, conveying that she felt understood. When she finished speaking, I asked her to lie down on the low Feldenkrais table in her most comfortable position. She chose to lie on her back, so I placed cushions under her head and knees to reduce unnecessary muscular effort. I sat next to her on a stool, where it was easy to maintain eye contact, and said: "I'm going to place my hands gently on the right side of your torso. Please let me know if something feels especially supportive. Using your attention this way trains your brain to notice and sense support. Your nervous system will learn to gravitate toward comfort, and to develop a soothing connection with yourself and others. Anytime you would like to pause, please let me know." This put Sally in charge, safely opening her up for new experiences. As I moved her slowly and predictably, she learned to trust herself and me. Our relationship became the training ground for her sensory, emotional, and movement reorganization. Monitoring and modifying sensorimotor responses was creating new synaptic connections in her brain.

I sensed her neurophysiological responses. My hands gently followed her breathing and fully connected with her right side, taking over the muscular contractions in her torso, inducing even muscular tonus throughout her body. Movement began to take place in every direction, like ripples in a pond.

Subtle movement reached toward her spine, chest, and up to her head; and she breathed more fully. I placed her right hand on her right lower ribs so she could sense herself. Touching the right side first activates the left hemisphere of the brain, providing the opportunity to integrate feelings without becoming overwhelmed. Making contact with the left side of the body first intensifies sensation and feelings. The sensorimotor system and mirror neurons are primarily in the right hemisphere. Sometimes I prefer to touch the left side first. Understanding the brain helps the practitioner design each *Functional Integration* (FI) session uniquely for the student's needs. After touching just the right side, I removed my hands and asked her what she was noticing, at which she smiled and said, "My right side feels bigger; at ease; even more present than the left." When I asked her whether she preferred her right or left side, she said, "The right side. The left feels crumpled and small. Will you make me even?"

"Yes," I said, "we will integrate all of you, in this easy, gentle way. This process is changing your mind map, your self-image. You are learning to experience your whole self in safe, new ways."

She laughed, "Maybe I *do* like feelings and sensations. I realize I have been struggling, but I didn't know I was doing so. I think I was afraid." Then tears rolled from her eyes. "I feel so relieved," she said.

I stayed next to her, leaving my hand on her forearm as she shared her experience, sensing her emotions changing as she naturally integrated. Her smile, laughter, and tears transformed into a calm, neutral state. Allowing the ebb and flow of sensations and emotions promotes open flow toward integration. I said, "You are learning the ability to self-regulate and to co-regulate. It's kind of like slow dancing." Open, adaptable, energized, and connected to others, we resonate, we feel calm. Sally sat up feeling stable and at ease. Standing, she felt taller and grounded; walking was also easier.

Our minds gravitate toward a stable view of the world, whether it is true or not. Sally's unexamined mindset about herself represented beliefs that ran her life and negatively affected her emotions, sensations, thoughts, and relationships. Feldenkrais helped her to shift her state, allowing her to challenge, change, integrate, and function at higher levels. The state shift that occurred while she was lying on the table immediately transferred to practical, usable daily functions, effortless and easy to remember.

As novelty increases learning, I made each lesson with Sally a little different. Once she remarked, "I feel grounded like a bear!" Another time, "I feel as free as a butterfly with movable wings." The pain in her hips, shoulders, and neck subsided as she learned to move efficiently. This lesson and many more helped Sally reach her goal. With practice, the new state will become a trait. This actually changes our self-image: the way we define ourselves, our beliefs about what we can and can't do. Comfortable sensations and freedom of movement become coupled with pleasant images. We can't undo the past, but with awareness we can integrate our feelings, sensations, thoughts, and actions; and when we do so, life transforms.

Skillful state shifting

Skillful state shifting is an important aspect of neurological change. A state is psychophysiological

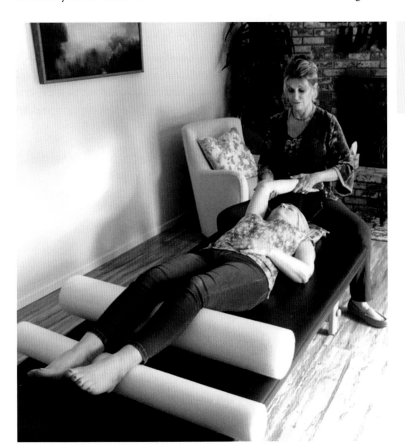

Figure 12.1
Donna Ray giving a *Functional Integration* lesson.

Courtesy of Donna Ray

and includes sensations, emotions, thoughts, and musculoskeletal movement organization, as well as the meaning attribute. Systems are interwoven; changing one aspect of a state changes the whole organism. The notion of changing the whole by changing a part is founded on dynamic systems theory (DST), a theoretical approach to the study of development that refers to systems of elements that change over time. DST evolved out of research on complex systems in fields like physics and mathematics but also incorporates thinking about systems in biology, psychology, and other disciplines. DST addresses the process of change and development, rather than specific developmental outcomes, and offers a set of concepts that helps us examine overall patterns of change, including stabilization, destabilization, and self-regulation (Thelen and Smith 1996).

Imagine the vastness of multiple systems inseparably functioning simultaneously: the vestibular system, located in the inner ear and involved with motion, head position, balance, and spatial orientation; the autonomic nervous system; the limbic system; the visual/ocular system; the digestive system; the bilateral brain system; the vertical information system; the social-play system; the sensorimotor system; and many more, automatically interacting. In addition, Dr Feldenkrais asserted that we have a reflex reaction system – a fear of falling – that is perceived physiologically as well as emotionally and mentally. Imagine tripping off a curb and almost falling: the stomach muscles tighten and the head tucks forward, preparing us for safe falling. This automatic protection pattern keeps us safe when falling, but when we contract and hold repeatedly, the neurophysiological anxiety pattern becomes problematic. The neck, chest, stomach, and hip flexors remain contracted, breathing is shallow, emotional and physical discomfort become chronic.

With skillful state shifting, these difficulties change at once, because they are interconnected as a whole pattern. In his book *The Elusive Obvious*, Feldenkrais (2019) describes this phenomenon in detail. Understanding this principle helps us comprehend how state shifting and altering movement patterns interrupt anxiety, stress, and trauma. Perhaps most importantly, the interruption is made and a new, more effective state is learned. Removing a pattern without providing an alternative one is not useful, and can even be destabilizing.

Remember, "All sensory and motor experience is accompanied by emotional expression; and that voluntary muscular patterns corresponding to these emotions are preceded by sensory experience… To every state there corresponds a pattern of muscular contraction" (Feldenkrais 2019). Emotion is arousal or excitation in your nervous system. The sensations come instantaneously and the mind quickly deciphers the excitation. Thoughts quickly interpret your sensation and emotions based on past experiences. *Awareness* interrupts the assumption and an alternative can be chosen.

Fear and anxiety are… seen to be the sensation of impulses arriving at the central nervous system from the organs and viscera… all emotions are connected with excitations arriving at the vegetative or autonomic nervous system or arising from the organs, muscles, etc. that it innervates. The arrival of such impulses to the higher centers of the central nervous system is sensed as emotion.

Feldenkrais 2019

Thought habits maintain categories; emotional excitation is placed in a belief category that has been constructed by past events, cultural mores, and family of origin experiences. When belief categories remain unexamined, they are maintained as truth, becoming pillars as solid as the Greek Parthenon. The self-image, or personality, is supported

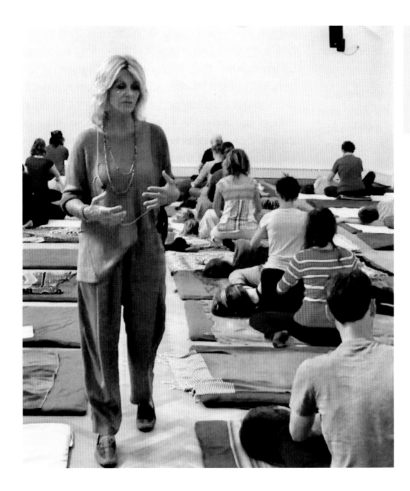

Figure 12.2
Donna Ray teaching an *Awareness Through Movement* class in Vienna, Austria.

Courtesy of Donna Ray

by these pillars, so strong that we take them for granted, fight for them, even kill to maintain them. By changing your neuromuscular patterns, your emotional thought patterns are changed as well. By shining a light on your beliefs, you synergistically heighten new ways of thinking, creating choices in your plane of possibilities.

Reducing anxiety through movement awareness

Dr Feldenkrais stated:

You are as good as you wish; you are certainly more creative in imagining alternatives than you know. If you know what you are doing and even more important 'how' you use yourself to act, you will be able to do things the way you want. I believe the world's most important advice, 'know thyself,' was first said by one who learned to know oneself.

Feldenkrais 2019

This integrative learning process changes how present thought and action take place, how the past is remembered, and in addition, it alters the imagined future. Anxiety relates to the imagined future, depression the remembered past. Reactions to the past and to an imagined future create stress physically, emotionally, and mentally. Stress, strain, and tension can be generated by the demands of adverse circumstances, or by the focus of attention toward the imagined past or future.

Getting ready to go on a flight is a common scenario for many. Calm, frequent flyers may give very little thought to travel. They may simply pack their suitcases and passports and download their travel itineraries. They don't imagine flight delays, disastrous crashes, turbulence, or lost luggage. Or, if they do, they have solutions for potential problems. In contrast, anxious, stressed flyers ruminate about negative past experiences or scary stories they have heard from others, creating fear and physical tension. The dread spills over into daily life, even before the travel begins. When the flight is over they are relieved, but anxiety over flying home may spoil the vacation.

Let's apply the Feldenkrais Method to this circumstance. The method asks us to slow down, to become aware of sensation, the physical relationship to thoughts and feelings. Frequently, tension in the neuromuscular system manifests as a tight jaw, neck, shoulders, low back. Shallow breathing and insomnia are typical anxiety, stress, and fear patterns. Feldenkrais practitioners train people to sense and feel moment to moment without judgment, without willfully trying to change. Awareness itself *creates* change. We advise: Slow down your movement a little bit. During sitting, standing, and walking, notice your breathing and exhale fully (this prompts the activation of the parasympathetic nervous system). See your surroundings, instilling feelings of safety and keeping you from imagining past or future. We harness attention by focusing on what is actually happening in our environment, emphasizing sensory stimuli, seeing, and hearing as well as movement sensations.

Awareness Through Movement (ATM) practice inherently emphasizes the above-mentioned suggestions. Small, gentle, pain-free movements create comfort and reorganize the nervous system. Utilization of this sensory bottom-up intervention, as opposed to a cognitive top-down approach, impacts our *interoception*: the sense of the internal state of the body. Deciphering the internal state of the body provides us with useful information; this awareness informs the choices that we make.

Practicing self-regulation

An easy way to shift our sensory state is tuning into exhalation, lengthening it. This shifts the autonomic nervous system toward the parasympathetic state of calmness and relaxation. Focusing on inhalation excites the nervous system and can intensify anxiety. As you are reading this, notice yourself exhaling fully. Sense your feet on the ground. Move your attention to your lower legs, your thighs, hips, pelvis. Sense the breath in your belly, back, chest, shoulders, neck, and head. Imagine all the parts in detail, then move your attention back down to your feet. You can also try scanning: close your eyes; notice your eyes moving as your attention shifts downward. Your sensorimotor system in the right hemisphere is now activated. Thoughts slow down, the sense of safety increases, it's easier to pay attention. Practice this anywhere, anytime, to interrupt a state of anxiety.

Along with scanning, we can add movements that further break up old habits in the neuromuscular system. After scanning as you just did, while sitting, lying down, or standing, gently look right and left. Observe yourself as you simply look right and left. Most people make a small movement of their head with their eyes. Each eye is connected to the right and left hemisphere. Moving your eyes right and left immediately alters your brain's processes, breaking up patterns of anxiety and stress. EMDR (eye movement desensitization and reprocessing), developed by Francine Shapiro, is a psychotherapeutic treatment that relies on the capacity to shift states solely via eye movement, a method I have utilized in my practice for 20 years (Shapiro 2017). Dr Feldenkrais created many ATM lessons that utilize eye movement as a source of state shifting and functional improvement. Next time you move your eyes to the right, move your left shoulder forward. Notice that your right shoulder moves back at the same time. Now sense your chest responding. Repeat this sequence three or four times. Rest in the middle; move your eyes to the right and then to the left. Sense the difference. Repeat the movements to the left. Notice the difference in your movement capacity and your state shift. (This brief example of ATM is expanded in the audio version at the end of the chapter.)

Self-regulation is useful anytime we want to harness our attention and create a state shift. Being out of balance and not regulating well is uncomfortable. Dysregulation is experienced through anxiety, worry, perseveration, insomnia, and sometimes lethargy, as well as social isolation, sexual response issues, poor focusing, interference with learning, and avoidance of situations. Dan Siegel's *The Developing Mind* discusses dysfunctional emotional regulation patterns, even psychiatric disturbances, which can be viewed as disorders of self-regulation. For example, sometimes attention deficit disorder is actually dysregulation caused by trauma and stress. Lack of self-regulation perpetuates dread, anxiety, worry, and inattention (Siegel 2015).

Feldenkrais lessons create confidence, inner stability, and actual improved balance, which result in resilience and the capacity to recover from difficulties quickly. The lessons prime the nervous system for alert, calm, grounded experience. This effective, painless, easy approach tackles negative, painful ways of behaving. State shifting is part of each lesson both in ATM, verbally guided movements, and in *Functional Integration* hands-on work, or combined verbal direction and hands-on guided movements.

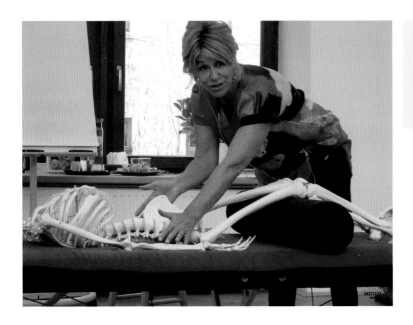

Figure 12.3
Donna Ray demonstrating on a skeleton in a Feldenkrais training program.

Courtesy of Donna Ray

ATM can be practiced alone, using audio, or in group classes. Individual sessions intensify learning. In my nearly 40 years of professional practice, I have found a combination of the above to be most effective. Feldenkrais practitioners steer away from diagnostic terms such as post-traumatic stress disorder, anxiety disorders, major depression, or attention deficit disorder. We do not diagnose pain or neurological disorders. But, as movement awareness guides, sensitive active listeners to verbal and non-verbal communication, we observe changes take place in behaviors related to these diagnostic categories. Feldenkrais practitioners are familiar with *neuroplasticity*: how the brain changes the mind and the mind changes the brain through movement and relationships (Doidge 2007).

Cultivating neutrality

ATM offers a variety of movement possibilities that are easy and pleasurable. These movements are gentle; they can be done routinely at home, in bed, in the line at the grocery store, lying on the floor in your living room, or sitting in your office. Doing them outdoors in nature, you will receive an added boost. You need no special equipment or outfits. Wherever you go, you have your own ability to move or imagine movement. These movements may fulfill your need to meditate while incorporating the benefits of pleasurable, restorative, functional movement.

Practicing Feldenkrais keeps us open, adaptive, energized, and resilient, because we are able to restore vitality and move well. Maintaining this way of being is possible by creating daily routines at home, listening to audible ATMs, attending weekly classes and/or workshops, and by visiting a Feldenkrais practitioner frequently or occasionally. The effect of the lessons creates what Dr Feldenkrais called a *tabula rasa*, a blank slate. A sense of neutrality is cultivated in ourselves that allows us to go in new directions, both physically and mentally. With this ability our lives become less rigid and chaotic. Fundamentally, we cannot control life events, but we feel capable and prepared to face life's challenges. We enjoy and embrace day-to-day moments: the breeze in the trees, the sun on our skin, the smile of a loved one. In calm, open states, we can savor the beauty that life offers.

References

Doidge, N. 2007. *The Brain that Changes Itself: Stories of personal triumph from the frontiers of brain science*, p. 42. Viking Books, New York.

Feldenkrais, M. 2019. The Body Pattern of Anxiety. *The Elusive Obvious*. Reprint edn., North Atlantic Books/ Somatic Resources, San Francisco, CA.

Shapiro, F. 2017. *Eye Movement Desensitization and Reprocessing (EMDR) Therapy: Basic Principles, Protocols, and Procedures*, 3rd edn. Guilford Press, New York, NY.

Siegel, D. 2015. *The Developing Mind*. Guilford Press, New York, NY.

Thelen, E., Smith, L.B. 1996. *A Dynamic Systems Approach to the Development of Cognition and Action*. MIT Press, Cambridge, MA.

Awareness Through Movement
Audio Lessons taught by Donna Ray

12.1 *Reducing Stress and Anxiety (Turning)*

12.2 *Reducing Stress and Anxiety (Sliding Hands)*

12.3 *Reducing Stress and Anxiety (Tilting)*

"She's got that creative touch."

"We need a creative solution to this issue."

"I like to call myself a cultural creative."

When you think "creative," often a person you know comes into mind: perhaps it's you, or someone you admire. What defines creativity and, really, what good is it? The answer at first seems obvious. Creative people create innovations that shift the world. They produce art that touches our emotions. They challenge the mundane and offer a window into new possibilities. Yet you can also probably name creative people who are unhappy, or use their creativity to create chaos, or even employ creative strategies for less than noble ends (like tax evasion, for example).

So, we have two challenges: first accessing creativity, and then making creativity functional. I've been exploring this theme probably since my first childhood attempt to build a mud city in the backyard didn't turn out so well. Great ideas need applied intelligence in order to yield the desired results.

Creativity is not simply talent. According to Moshe Feldenkrais (2010, p. 180), talent is not something you are born with, but something that you learn. So, creativity is not a gift but a result. A creative act is actually a process. In many ways, this process is analogous to a Feldenkrais *Awareness Through Movement* (ATM) or *Functional Integration* lesson. The student has a curiosity and a desire to explore and improve their relationship to self-image. It could involve a problem or a challenge: recovering from an injury, getting past a stuck place in performance, or overcoming other perceived limitations. The blank canvas, the musical obstacle, or the plot twist offers another kind of challenge. But

creativity is not just for the arts: problems and difficulties abound in politics, business, and science. Creativity is a process for improving and solving all of life's challenges: from the boardroom to the family room.

In both a Feldenkrais lesson and a life challenge, a creative person begins with a self-assessment. An actor, for example, may say: "I'm 35 years old and the character I'm playing is 45. What are the differences? The actress playing opposite me has an attitude: she seems to think that she is the lead and is treating me like some extra. I wonder if I need to do some research into what was going on in 1945 when the play takes place?" In a Feldenkrais lesson, the student begins with observing: "What is my contact with the floor like? Where am I comfortable, or uncomfortable? What are the differences between my right and left shoulder blades? I see that I still feel a bit shaky from that near accident on the way to class."

Both processes begin with noticing what's available, what's uncomfortable, and what is moving. Then comes exploration of the possible: "What if we try this? How does that feel? Where does it feel stuck?" In a Feldenkrais lesson, this takes place through movement. But the same questions apply when beginning to write, dance, or run a meeting.

Feldenkrais learning principles form the core of the creative process. Madelyn Kent is a Guild Certified Feldenkrais Practitioner and the creator of Sense Writing, which provides training for writers that integrates ATM with the creative writing process. One of the principles in her course is paradox. One of the most powerful paradoxes in Feldenkrais learning is the principle that *less is more*. Instead of trying to force more movement from an injured

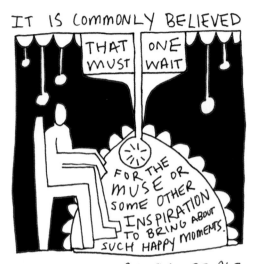

IT IS COMMONLY BELIEVED

THAT MUST ONE WAIT

FOR THE MUSE OR SOME OTHER INSPIRATION TO BRING ABOUT SUCH HAPPY MOMENTS.

BUT MATURE, CREATIVE PEOPLE HAVE LEARNED TO KNOW THEMSELVES SUFFICIENTLY WELL SO THAT THEY CAN BRING THEMSELVES TO THE REVERSIBLE STATE OF ACTURE.

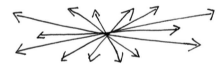

Figure 13.1
"It is commonly believed that one must wait for the muse…" Quote from Moshe Feldenkrais 2002. *The Potent Self: A Study of Spontaneity and Compulsion.* North Atlantic Books, Berkeley, CA, p. 199.

Courtesy of Tiffany Sankary 2014. *Feldenkrais Illustrated: The Art of Learning.* Movement and Creativity Press, Somerville, MA

arm, obsessing over the musical passage that won't reveal itself, or painting and re-painting the image that refuses to manifest, one can harness the entire nervous system by working somewhere else, or in a different way. Kent (2017) wrote:

Ruthy Alon writes in Mindful Spontaneity *(1996): 'When movement is difficult, you are entitled to the assistance of various compromises, such as partial movement, all kinds of supporting pads, rhythm change, activation from another direction, assistance from another part of your body.' All of these have their corollaries in Sense Writing. If for example, a writer finds herself stuck, she might write into scenes that take place just minutes before or after the 'problematic' scene and go deeply into those moments, though they were never part of 'the story.'*

Another paradox is what some practitioners call "an investment in failure." This is a willingness to make mistakes, to fail, and to allow oneself to be okay with being confused. If one remembers that both creativity and a Feldenkrais lesson are a process, then mistakes become part of that learning process. Moshe Feldenkrais (1985, p. 179) said, "Making mistakes is essential to satisfactory learning." Indeed, while trying to make my mud city, I learned that filling Mom's good water glasses with mud and trying to bang the mud out not only didn't work, but it resulted in broken glass, cut fingers, and scolding. This led me in other creative directions that I wouldn't have tried if my first experiment had been successful.

Uri Vardi, a cellist, Feldenkrais teacher, and professor at the University of Wisconsin–Madison, encourages his students to interrupt their habitual striving by exaggerating their mistakes. "Instead of correcting, I will instruct them to aim at the same place (on the cello) that they miss. Now aim at missing that note. Really miss it, exactly to where you miss it. Once you have the ability to miss it well, you have the ability to do anything" (Feldenkrais Awareness Summit 2019). This strategy frees the student to stop "trying" and allows the music, or the dance step, or the Feldenkrais movement, to be discovered from another angle. After all, if it wasn't for mistakes, we wouldn't have Post-it® Notes.

Tiffany Sankary is an artist, a Feldenkrais Assistant Trainer, and the author of the book *Feldenkrais Illustrated.* Speaking about her creative process, she wrote: "Confusion keeps me searching for what's next and what's needed. I look for what to get rid of, what's extraneous. I listen for the poetry and the moments of grace. It is not always clear and then there are moments when it is" (Sankary 2017). Similarly, in a Feldenkrais lesson one attends to habitual holdings, or, as Moshe Feldenkrais called them, "parasitic habits." These *extraneous* tensions or ways of moving can prevent the experience of grace. The permission to not know, to be confused, to fail, to not strive for success, allow creativity a place to flourish. Fear of failure stifles many creative impulses. When we give ourselves permission to make a mistake, or two, or a dozen, we open the door to seeing different possible outcomes to our efforts.

Alan Questel, a Feldenkrais Trainer, suggests in his book, *Creating Creativity* (out of print but Kindle edition available), that an essential aspect of creativity is choice. To be able to choose among options, perhaps to even create options in a given situation, is a creative act. "The simple answer is that the creative person understands choice. They know how to create choices. They know how to make choices" (Questel 2000).

Let's take a break from all this thinking and look at how some of these principles are explored through movement. You are probably reading this in a book or on an e-reader, so we'll do something in sitting. Come to the front edge of your seat and place both feet flat on the floor. Have you already interrupted your habitual way of doing something? How does that feel? Notice your thoughts. Is this comfortable or uncomfortable for you? Now lift one foot and put it on top of your head.

What?

Notice how you felt when you read that sentence. There are a whole range of responses one could make – from actually trying it, to scoffing at the absurdity of it. Trying to put your foot on your head in one go could be the equivalent of trying to

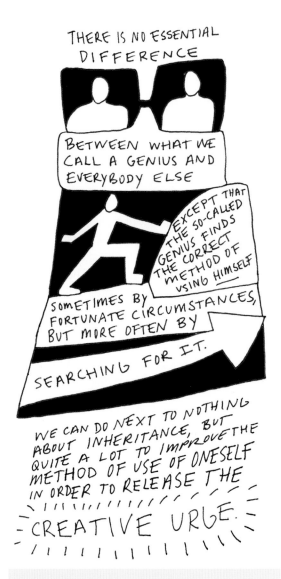

Figure 13.2

"There is no essential difference between what we call a genius and everybody else..." Quote from Moshe Feldenkrais 2002. *The Potent Self: A Study of Spontaneity and Compulsion*. North Atlantic Books, Berkeley, CA, p. 3.

Courtesy of Tiffany Sankary 2014. *Feldenkrais Illustrated: The Art of Learning*. Movement and Creativity Press, Somerville, MA compose an orchestral masterpiece. Now of course, you may be a yogi, or acrobat, so putting your foot on your head is no big deal. But then ask yourself, do you always put your foot on your head in the same way? Is there an easier way to put your foot on your head while sitting in a chair?

You may have encountered this quote from Feldenkrais already: "Making the impossible possible, the possible easy, and the easy elegant." Each of us begins a project or a movement from where we are.

Our problem or challenge may seem like a silly one: putting the foot on top of the head. But it's no more foolish than wishing to write the great American novel or creating a memorable painting. The poet Rumi once said, "Start a huge, foolish project like Noah… it makes absolutely no difference what people think of you" (Rumi 1988). The beauty of the Feldenkrais Method is that it offers a way to do the impossible, by starting with what's easy. And in an ATM lesson, there is no one to judge you for trying something silly.

So how do we begin to apply Feldenkrais' principles of learning to creative solutions? We begin by exploring what is available. Instead of continuing to just try to force, push, and stretch the foot up, try the following:

1 Interlace your fingers and place them behind your head – not the neck, but the back of your skull. Lower your head and allow your elbows to drop. Think of the weight of your head (11 lbs/5 kg) yielding to gravity. Your elbows point downward toward your thighs. Let your head keep going down, as if you wanted to kiss your navel (another impossible move, although it might be fun to try it).

   Notice: Are you breathing? Do you exhale or inhale as you do it? Which one is easier? Make a creative choice and find out for yourself. What do you feel in your spine? Can your chest soften? Let your pelvis and hips roll

back. Can you feel the sit bones change their relationship to the chair?

So much is going on in a moment of lowering the head. If you add noticing your thoughts and emotions, you could just lower your head all day.

Instead, sit back and take a rest.

In any creative process, it's important to pause. Whether that pause is a short walk, a cup of tea, or even doing a Feldenkrais lesson, you need to literally step away from your task to allow your system to process the work you have done. Return to the front of the chair as before. Check in. Is your sitting different? Let's explore a paradox. Begin doing the same movement you were doing – lowering your head with your hands interlaced behind your head, your back rounding, your elbows down. When you get to your lowest point, still holding your head, point your elbows forward and then begin reaching them toward the ceiling. It's as if someone in front of you took hold of your elbows so that they make a kind of scoop, then whoosh up toward the ceiling. So now it's like a circle of sorts: you lower your head rounding your back, then scoop up and arch your back. When you arch your back, you are moving *away* from your stated goal (foot on head) and yet you are holding your intention of putting your foot on your head.

Think back to Madelyn Kent's strategy of writing "around the scene."

Rest.

2 Come forward in your chair again. Begin to slide your right hand down the outside of your right leg toward your foot. Down and up several times. Repeat on the inside of your leg (Figure 13.3). Try the same thing with your left

hand and your left leg. Now have some fun. Slide your right hand down your left leg. You choose: inside or outside. Explore. Changing hands, including the original moves, turn it into your own chair sliding dance.

Notice (while you're busy having fun): What does your head do? Look down? Turn? Do you have a choice? Are you breathing? Is one side easier than the other? Do you have an attitude of needing to reach your foot? If you can't reach your foot, are you judging yourself? ("Damn, I'm so inflexible.") Notice that, as you are moving, you are also sensing, feeling, and thinking. When you've had enough,

rest. Can you see that in a somatic way, this was a creative process? You made choices constantly: which arm, how far to go, where to place your head, etc.

3 Interlace your fingers behind your right thigh and lower your head toward it (Figure 13.4). Now, keeping that same distance between your head and thigh, lift your leg. Of course, this is virtually impossible, unless you let yourself "roll" backwards. As you lift your leg, lean back, but *don't* lift your head! Simply let yourself have fun picking up your leg and leaning back in your chair. Just don't go so far

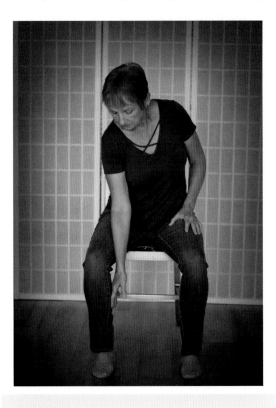

Figure 13.3
Slide the right hand down the inside of the right leg.

Courtesy of Ron Morecraft

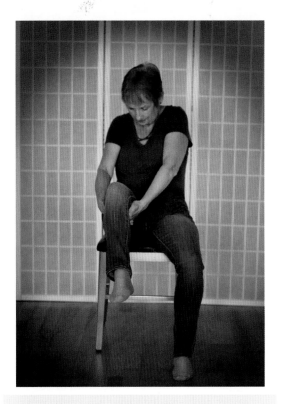

Figure 13.4
Link the fingers of both hands behind the right thigh and lift, lowering the head.

Courtesy of Ron Morecraft

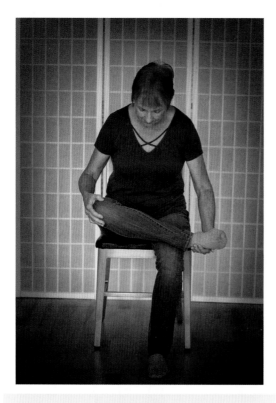

Figure 13.5
Cross the right ankle over the left thigh, holding the knee with the right hand and the foot with the left hand.

Courtesy of Ron Morecraft

that you put yourself off balance. Try it with your other leg.

Notice: What is the shape of your back? When do you exhale? Do you feel safe? Silly? Curious?

4 If this movement feels impossible, or you have severe problems with your hip joints, you can skip it. You've done plenty already. Part of our learning process is also knowing when enough is enough for us. I can't tell you how many times I've injured myself in my life because I

needed to pull just one more weed, trim one more piece of tile, reach up to one more shelf. Honor your body's intelligence.

If, however, you are having a great time, lift your right leg and cross your ankle over your left thigh. Grab your knee with your right hand and your foot with your left. Bend your head toward your shin (Figure 13.5).

Here comes the part when you do something utterly mad. There comes a point in the creative process where you just have to try something different.

Jimi Hendrix kissed the sky. You just have to kiss your shin. From the knee to the ankle, just reach your head and mouth in little pecks, as if you were eating an ear of corn, up and down your shin. Don't worry if you don't reach your shin, it's another impossible thought. Then put your leg down and rest. When you feel ready, try the other leg.

Digression: Playing, exploring, letting go of the need for a result; this is what we did as children. Through that process came discoveries and new learning. When we let go of the linear thinking process and expand our thinking in other directions, new insights and even solutions can appear. Some people call this redirecting of attention lateral thinking or thinking outside the box.

So now, we return to the original intention. Grab a foot and put it on your head. Maybe by this time, you really don't care if your foot reaches your head, because you've learned so many other things about yourself. Perhaps, to your surprise, your foot actually goes there. Or maybe you have discovered a whole new way to reach your foot.

You are actually creating at every moment as you cultivate your self-image. You are creating your relationship to others, to yourself, and so much more. The trick, as Moshe Feldenkrais said so often, is to actually know that you are doing it.

You've learned how artists apply Feldenkrais principles to their creative process. You've experienced a Feldenkrais lesson that illustrates these same creative strategies. There is still one tremendous benefit for enhancing the creative process: the Feldenkrais lessons themselves. MaryBeth Smith was a Feldenkrais practitioner, singer, and writer who worked extensively with performers, helping them connect ATM lessons with their creative process. She said:

The Feldenkrais Method has given me an almost-foolproof creativity catalyst. It is the question, "What else could I do?" In other words, what's another way to lift my foot? Maybe not so high this time; maybe slower; maybe on a different trajectory... Suddenly I am initiating endless variations on my way to a solution or product. And I know that one or more of those variations will work. That confidence in the iterative process makes me eager to 'be creative' again and again in other settings. My self-image changes from the inside out: I am creative.

Smith, personal communication March 2019

When you let go of your tasks and engage in a somatic learning experience, you are bringing together thinking, sensing, feeling, and movement into new ways of being. There are other chapters in this book that address the neurological processes taking place; here one can simply say, when you have writer's block, lie down and do an ATM lesson. You may be surprised at the result.

In the words of Moshe Feldenkrais:

Only when in possession of the full range of functioning on each level or plane of action can we eliminate compulsion to the degree that our action becomes the expression of our spontaneous selves. All creative men and women know spells when they can act in this manner.

Feldenkrais 1985, p. 199

References

Feldenkrais, M. 1985. *The Potent Self.* Harper & Row, San Francisco, CA.

Feldenkrais, M. 2010. Movement and the mind, interview with Will Schutz. In: E. Beringer (ed.) *Embodied Wisdom: The collected papers of Moshe Feldenkrais*, pp. 179–189. North Atlantic Books, Berkeley, CA.

Kent, M. 2017. An Introduction to Sense Writing, or Life, I Thought, Was Harder Than That. *Feldenkrais Journal* 30:46.

Questel, A. 2000. *Creating Creativity*, p. 10. Available from Uncommonsensing.com

Rumi 1988. *We Are Three*. Translated by Barks, C. Maypop, Athens, GA.

Sankary, T. 2017. "Confusion and Creativity." www.movementandcreativity.com/blog/podcast/confusionandcreativity [Accessed October 2020].

Finding My Middle *Awareness Through Movement* Audio Lesson taught by Lavinia Plonka

14A   Behind the Music   *Andrew Gibbons*

I once brought a pair of binoculars to a Martha Argerich concert. As a young musician, her recordings had left me both exhilarated and awed. It was a rare opportunity to see the pianist perform live. My seat was near the back of the hall, and so I smuggled in the extra magnification. But there was nothing to see. The binoculars only confirmed my ignorance. Whether trilling at a whisper, thundering with octaves, or weaving complex passage work, Argerich's kaleidoscopic sound emanated from a simple contact with the keys. It was like watching a sleight of hand artist, where stupefying effects are produced, yet the means of production are camouflaged. In everything, she hid the work.

Over the past 17 years in my career as a Feldenkrais practitioner in New York City, I've had the good fortune to work with musicians who play in the upper echelons of classical, jazz, and pop music: string players, pianists, singers, clarinetists, harpists, conductors, bassists, and drummers. And for the past ten years, I've spent a week each summer working with elite musicians at the Marlboro Music Festival in Brattleboro, VT.

To the outside observer, musicians at this level hide their work very well. But the pursuit of competent expression on an instrument does not exempt them from wear, tear, and injury. The complexity of the repertoire, the repetitive nature of practice, the constraints of the instrument, and the rigor of so much focus on the dexterity of the small muscles can come at a cost. Aches, pains, and sometimes full-blown injuries are inevitable. Careers are dimmed or are sometimes cut short. The great

American pianist and teacher Leon Fleisher, who crippled his right hand with a piano technique that married finger strain to musical expression, said, "Musicians are small muscle athletes" (Fleisher 2008). But Fleisher's quote risks misinterpretation, because while the *overwork* of these small muscles is often highlighted by their injuries, these muscles neither perform in a vacuum nor are they the proper locus of concern if musical expression is to flourish and have longevity. The dexterous small muscles are supported by a massive background of muscular, skeletal, and vestibular resources – an entire perceptual gestalt. Divorcing the effort at the periphery from the active support of this background is a reliable recipe for injury, though it may take time to fully bake.

The elements of musical intention – the movements, perceptions, thoughts, and emotions – are both filtered through and built upon a stubborn, though reliable, background of muscular habit: what is often called *posture*.

But a comprehensive training of this dynamic whole – posture as the basis for action and perception – is rarely well integrated into a musician's curriculum. Most musicians, as they construct their competency at an instrument, are prescribed exercises and études where they woodshed certain technical aspects to gain strength. Others find that learning the pieces in the repertoire itself provides them with the technical foundation they need. But these approaches remain both instrument-specific and downstream of the more foundational problem of posture and its relationship to action.

Writer Matias Dalsgaard describes the problem in this passage about the "Insecure Overachiever":

Such a person must have no stable or solid foundation to build upon. And yet tries to build his way out of the problem. It is an impossible situation. You can't compensate for having a foundation made of quicksand by building a new story on top of it. But this person takes no notice and hopes the problem down in the foundations won't be found out, if only the construction work keeps on going.

Dalsgaard, cited in Brooks 2019

When the foundations of posture are well organized with the periphery, the dexterity and capacity of the small muscles are not only greater and safer, but they coexist in a framework of mutual support and feedback.

The Feldenkrais Method puts this relationship front and center and asks you to look directly into this blind spot. How can you learn to play well not *in spite* of what you do with the rest of your body, but *because* of it?

This process of training a person to hone their entire cognitive and perceptual capacity toward a more perfect harmony in action – this is the aim of the Feldenkrais Method. And *Awareness Through Movement*, the self-directed modality within the work, is the best description of its goal and its path.

Awareness is the cognitive resource that allows a person to discriminate the essential effort from the superfluous, the cross-motivated, and the potentially harmful. And it is best trained in a rigorous context of experiment, testing, and discovery. Instead of teaching magic movements or prescriptive exercise, the Feldenkrais Method uses movement as the context for refining the internal image of skillful action. The idea is to both question and edit the very foundation of action so that our artistic expression actually has a healthy future.

The Feldenkrais Method offers musicians several advantages in this regard.

An intelligent retreat from performance

"If a passerby can recognize the song being played, it's not being practiced correctly," according to a rule of thumb at the Meadowmount School of Music (Coyle 2009).

Musicians understand the necessity of practice. But any musician who has logged these countless domain-specific hours knows that they can be fraught with disorganized effort and a compulsive striving toward what the writer Bill Zinsser calls "the tyranny of the final product" (Zinsser 2013). The Feldenkrais context offers an intelligent retreat from performance mode, where a musician can train the instrument that plays the instrument. By training the nervous system to make finer discriminations, students engage with the kind of experiments where deep, lasting learning can take root, and where their passive assumptions about how the body works are replaced with active literacy. Feldenkrais does this through several basic strategies designed to increase the caliber of attention, emphasize safety, and foster creativity.

Permission to slow down

Students are encouraged to go sufficiently slowly for their attention to the aesthetic details of movement to become easier. This pace allows them to sense where their muscles engage smoothly, where things get stiff or stuck, where they hold their breath, where the eyes become fixed or strained – and then shows them what to do about it. Without this pacing, a person will only tend to reenact their muscular habits of achievement, and there is no actual discovery, no new specificity. It is only through the quieting down of the habitual muscular and cognitive habits that an editing process, and a choice of more desirable behavior, can emerge.

Refinement over repetition

The concept of repetition, as in typical exercise, is eschewed. Instead, within the explorations of a certain movement, the student uses these iterations for refinement. One version of this is to taper each iteration closer and closer to the point of initiation of the movement, where the roots of many habits can be seen. Students who follow this advice discover that there is almost no end to the improvement they can create.

Use of constraints

Constraints in practicing (hands separately, playing only the chords, working a particular measure, singing the bass while playing the melody) allow a musician to break down the aspects of a composition so they can be stabilized in the ear, honed, and then integrated with other aspects of the music.

The Feldenkrais Method also uses constraints to help a person move away from the fiction of adopting better posture, and presuming a consequent benefit, toward the detailed work of investigating the rich and beautiful relationships the brain relies upon to compose movement.

The aim is to illuminate sensations and foster connections often hidden by their history of muscular habit. Constraints not only help to illuminate these connections, they also teach someone to be inventive and creative as they learn to integrate the many parts of their body in action.

For example:

- *Constraints of orientation*: Keeping the eyes on the horizon while moving from sitting to lying;

- *Constraints of initiation*: Reversing the proximal distal relationship (moving the arms relative to the spine versus moving the spine relative to the arms);

- *Constraints of perception*: Making movements on one side of the body while imagining them on the other;

- *Constraints of attention*: Measuring ankle movements via the changing tones of the neck muscles;

- *Constraints of timing*: Closing the hand so that all five fingers touch at the same moment.

Constraints deny a person the ability to move according to their habit. They enforce rigorous attention within the uncertainty by emphasizing particular criteria. In order to orient within a new standard, old patterns must be inhibited, new ones formed, and the student learns how to untie the knot of their personal history and posture.

Safe by design

Dr Feldenkrais was a fierce advocate of avoiding the neurological noise and psychological frustration of employing effort for its own sake.

Because of its emphasis on learning and discrimination, much of the Feldenkrais curriculum is safe by design. The lessons cultivate an ethos of patience, curiosity, and minimal effort to enhance sensation.

There are more challenging lessons, of course, using larger transitions and faster, sometimes ballistic movements. But the emphasis on specificity and discrimination make the work ideal for musicians who want to build a cognitive and physical foundation that will last and support their playing.

Strategic spaces

To enhance the internal image of posture, the Feldenkrais Method employs rests, suspensions of action, and pauses during the lessons. These create a balance between action and reflection, so the student becomes more adept at measuring and appreciating the kinesthetic changes and improvements that take place in the moment. For example, during the sit-to-stand process explored in the "What is Good Posture?" lesson in Moshe Feldenkrais' book *Awareness Through Movement*, you're instructed to interrupt the process of standing up, and to measure the in-between moments that make up the action, almost like stopping a film to examine each frame's composition. Feldenkrais (1972) wrote: "Halt the intention to get up, and see which part of the body relaxes as a result. This is the effort that was superfluous to correct getting up. This is not easy, and you'll have to pay close attention to detect it." More specifically, the superfluous effort is that which you can reduce while *still maintaining the length in your spine and your readiness to move*. Students often find that inhibiting one layer of effort reveals a more essential stability underneath it. This subtle internal game of editing your self-organization can seem painstaking and unusual, as most of us only measure the success of our attempts at the end. But it is a potent process-oriented tool, and I have seen it work to great effect for musicians who struggle with excessive tension as well as for those with longstanding difficulties and entrenched habits of playing.

The ability to support the length of the spine as you transition from one place to another has been a particular area of interest for me in my private practice. Pianists, for example, often need help connecting their pelvis effectively to their spine and arms, and often lose it in the transitions they make when they are away from the middle position at the keyboard. That they don't know they lose it, and keep playing anyway, is the real issue.

Over the years, I have seen very few pianists, including high-level artists, who have any criteria for this foundational aspect of their playing, or were ever shown the basics in this regard. They sit on the pelvis; but they do not *play* from it.

One of the tools I use with clients is a hard cardboard cylinder: a roller. Students spend time sitting on the roller and leaning toward and away from the piano. The roller helps in two ways:

1 It is unstable and forces the student to find a connection from the pelvis to the spine and move with this connection intact.

2 The roller provides a very narrow purchase for the student to find support for their pelvis and torso, forcing them immediately to become more specific in their aim and coordination from below as they move their arms at the instrument. This kind of *forced accuracy* is a

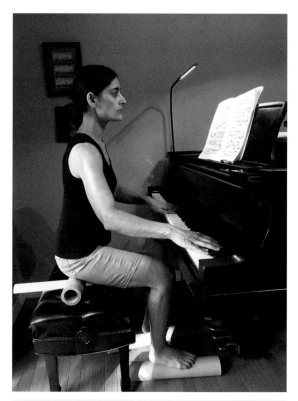

Figure 14.1
Sitting on a simple cardboard roller.

Courtesy of Andrew Gibbons

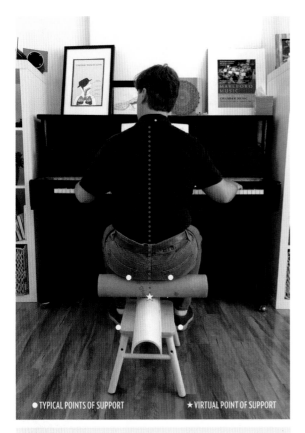

Figure 14.2
A more challenging roller on a half roller.

Courtesy of Andrew Gibbons

useful constraint, because, when combined with demonstration and an examination of some of the relevant bones, the student begins to form a functional image of this important hub to which some of the most powerful muscles in their body attach.

That the roller is unfamiliar in the beginning is not a problem, since the learning process is only mildly challenging and often reveals an aspect of the confusion under which the student developed their habits and injuries (Figure 14.1). As they

progress, I introduce them to even bigger constraints, like one roller perched upon another half-roller (Figure 14.2). The piling of unstable surfaces leads them to find the most precise, even, and central skeletal support that many of them have ever experienced, as the point of sustentation is directly beneath the spine. Explorations like this produce not only better kinesthetic and vestibular control but also introduce the student to a kind of creativity that can change their approach to solo practice time.

In the end, the maturation of an artist must be away from unconscious, compulsive action and toward the capacity for choice. This includes not only what to learn, but how to learn it. Every masterclass I've ever watched tended toward this particular refinement. The student plays, and the master helps them investigate the musical choices they made or failed to make, or weren't even aware of, and guides them in the way of making clearer, more specific choices in the piece.

Learning, as I see it, is not the training of willpower but the acquisition of the skill to inhibit parasitic action and the ability to direct clear motivations as a result of self-knowledge. It is perhaps not unconnected with this that all creative people do things in their own way. Painters, mathematicians, composers and everybody else who has ever done anything worthwhile, always had to learn to paint, think, and compose – but not in the way they were taught. They had to learn and work until they knew themselves sufficiently to bring themselves to the state of spontaneity in which their deepest inner self could be brought up and out. Such people are not free of compulsion – much to the contrary. The difference is that what they produce out of the state of compulsion has some value because of the true spontaneous nature of the production.

Moshe Feldenkrais (1998, p. xl)

References

Brooks, D. 2019. *The Second Mountain: The quest for a moral life*, p. 24. Random House, New York.

Coyle, D. 2009. *The Talent Code: Greatness isn't born. It's grown. Here's how*, pp. 84–85. Bantam, New York.

Feldenkrais, M. 1972. *Awareness Through Movement*. Harper and Row, New York.

Feldenkrais, M. 1998. *The Potent Self: A study of spontaneity and compulsion*. Reprint, Frog Books/Somatic Resources, Berkeley, CA.

Fleisher, L. 2008. "NPR Interview: Leah Fleisher Cures What Ails Musicians," https://text.npr.org/89408904 [Accessed November 2020]

Zinsser, W. 2013. *On Writing Well*, 30th Anniversary Edition, Ch. 22. Harper Collins, New York.

Lengthening the Armpits *Awareness Through Movement* Audio Lesson taught by Andrew Gibbons

14B   Voice/Singing   *Marina Gilman*

Introduction: What is voice?

Voice is the most somatic of all instruments. It is the source not only of verbal communication and singing, but of all the vegetative functions such as coughing, crying, and laughing. According to the Merriam-Webster online dictionary, the term *voice* describes the specific sound produced by vertebrates, in this case humans: a. "by means of lungs, larynx, or syrinx" [birds]; "b.(1) musical sound produced by the vocal folds and resonated by the cavities of the head and throat."[1]

These definitions suggest that voice, that is the sounds produced by the structures within the neck, are limited in some way to the head and neck. In reality, vocal production is of the whole body. The ease and function of the sounds we make are affected by how we stand, sit, breathe, and move. The height of the heels of our shoes, the tension in the jaw, neck, shoulders, and abdomen, as well as the position of the knees and feet all influence the quality, range, and resonance of our voices.

The importance of posture in voice training, whether for singing or acting, has long been stressed. The renowned vocal pedagogue, Manuel Garcia (1805–1906), credited with the development of the first laryngeal mirror, extolled the virtue of the "noble posture" for good singing. One of his younger contemporaries, G.B. Lamperti (1839–1910) suggested that "the position of the body must be easy and natural…" (2012, p. 3). More recently, singing teachers and speech-language pathologists LeBorgne and Rosenberg (2014, p. 3) stated, "Posture and alignment are among the foundational principles of good singing." Notably, the late acting voice coach Arthur Lessac (1997, p. 20) wrote, "The function of breathing determines the structure of posture at the very same time that the function of posture determines the structure of breathing."

It is in this realm of teaching the voice as an integral aspect of the body that the Feldenkrais Method can be a valuable tool in voice training, whether for singers, actors, teachers, preachers, or indeed anyone who desires to improve their voice. Feldenkrais trainer Alan Questel recalls a quote by the director Peter Brook: "The very base of the work of every actor is his own body – and nothing is more concrete… In [Feldenkrais] I have met someone with a scientific formation who possesses a global mastery of his subject. He has studied the body in movement with a precision that I found nowhere else" (Questel and St Cyr 1995).

To better understand the connections between the voice and the rest of the body, let us briefly review how human vocal sounds (phonation) are produced. In basic terms, the sound source is the vibration of the vocal folds generated by airflow up from the lungs. The vocal folds themselves are the internal structures of the larynx or voice box. Air from the lungs is then converted to sound waves by the vibration of the vocal folds. These sound waves resonate in the mouth, nose, bones, and tissue of the face and are in turn shaped by movements of the tongue, lips, and palate into the specific sounds we associate with speech and singing. The perceptual difference between speaking and singing is determined by resonance, that is, how we color the sounds, the range (both pitch and loudness), and the duration of syllables.

Vocal structures: somatic connections

The larynx is supported in the neck by muscles attached to the tongue, jaw, clavicle, shoulder girdle, back of the pharynx (throat), and sternum and sits on top of the trachea (windpipe). The anatomical vocal structures are in the neck, with the resonating chamber in the mouth. It is easy to understand that as the shape of the neck changes, such as by moving the head forward and backward, the sound of the voice alters. In fact, research studies have shown

that muscles of the shoulders and neck (sternocleidomastoid, scalene and trapezius, and muscles of the posterior neck) activate during phonation (Pettersen 2005; Watson, Williams, and James 2012). Since the power source for the phonation comes from the lungs, there is direct involvement of the ribcage, diaphragm, and abdominal muscles. We breathe differently depending on our task and our position in space. It is clear then that balance has a major influence on our ability to breathe effectively. For example, standing with knees locked tilts the pelvis in such a way as to tighten the abdominal muscles, which in turn restricts the ability of the diaphragm to easily contract. In other words, the whole skeletal structure is involved in optimal breathing and therefore vocal production (Kooijman et al. 2005).

One of the principles of the Feldenkrais Method, that force must travel *through* joints rather than across or around them, in order to avoid shearing forces, means that when this force is disrupted or diverted, phonation becomes less efficient and more effortful. With respect to voice, posturographic studies have shown voice changes in loudness and level of phonatory effort required (Giovanni, Akl, and Ouaknine 2008; Lagier et al. 2010; Nacci et al. 2012). A more recent study by Rollins (2017) found significant effects on the harmonic spectrum in singers between standing without shoes and with high heels related to postural changes.

Application of the Feldenkrais Method

Tension in the body and restricted breathing are paired. Releasing the breath can only happen when there is reduction of tension elsewhere in the body. Therefore, it makes sense that changes in breathing and increased coordination of movement throughout the body can improve vocal production. Many elements, both physiological and functional, are involved in efficient use of the breath in voice production. Posture is the most obvious of these elements. That is, posture not as generally defined in terms of standing or sitting rigidly but as a functional dynamic entity. Feldenkrais (1949, p. 74) defined proper posture as being a high level of ease of movement, consisting of three elements: the ability to: initiate movement in any direction with the same ease; start any movement without a preliminary adjustment; and move with the minimum of work, that is, with the maximum of efficiency.

With this in mind, the goal of Feldenkrais lessons is to help the individual discover through movement how their body can move with increased ease. With respect to breathing, there are as many ways to breathe as there are people on this earth. We breathe differently depending on our task – weightlifting versus singing; on our relationship to gravity – standing versus sitting or lying; on our emotional state – calm versus agitated. By the same token, there are many ways to teach breathing. So how do we learn to breathe effectively for singing or acting?

The lessons described below are from the collection of written and recorded lessons Feldenkrais taught in Tel Aviv. They are known as the Alexander Yanai lessons, referring to the location of his studio. These lessons exist in many variations as they are taught and transcribed by trainers and practitioners.

Moshe Feldenkrais only developed a few specific lessons that directly explore vocalization. The best known is "Equalizing the Nostrils" (Feldenkrais 1995, pp. 25–29). In this lesson he explores resonance by directing the air first through each nostril on the lowest tone, then highest tone on the vowel "ah." The lesson then continues, having the student speak a text in three variations: with the mouth closed normally, the mouth open but teeth closed, then the mouth and teeth closed. The changes in resonance can be remarkable. At the close of the lesson, he asks students to do a body scan to feel for changes in their breathing and how their body is lying differently. This lesson promotes optimization of airflow first through the nose, with the nasalized vowel "ah," then through the mouth with speaking text, and at the same time it uncouples the movement of the tongue from the jaw and lips, releasing tension in the tongue, jaw, and neck muscles.

Changes in breathing and resonance can be addressed in many ways. In "Touch the Floor in Standing," Feldenkrais (1995, pp. 2169–2176) draws attention to his own vocal quality in the simple act of bending to touch his knee and then gradually being able to touch the floor. He demonstrates how his voice changes:

> *If I do the movement like this, you feel it in my voice... In other words, breathing cannot take place without it being neutral. If the approach to movement is without neutrality... [incomplete sentence]. Before we try to improve the manner of expression, it is necessary that the skeleton – that means the essential part of the movement – will be clear, simple.*
>
> p. 2170

The primary activity of this lesson is bending to touch the knee and then the floor. However, the underlying focus is on finding ease of movement in the neck, shoulders, ribs, and spine, which in turn frees the breath and the voice. The lesson does not involve any vocalization. The movements are all directed to reaching down to touch the knee and eventually toward the floor. He begins bending forward to touch the knee, first with one arm then the other, and eventually both. Variations including turning the arm right and left; reaching to the back of the leg and to the side of the leg are added as the session progresses. The essence of the lesson has nothing to do with bending, but learning to release hidden tension in the back, chest, neck, and shoulders.

Case Study

John, a professional tenor, was singing four to six short shows a day for three consecutive days over the weekends at the Renaissance Faire. By Monday when he came for a lesson, he was very hoarse and barely able to sustain a sound. At the beginning of the "Equalizing the Nostrils" lesson it was difficult for him to phonate at any pitch. Gradually, he discovered how to let the air move through the nose without force, resulting in easier and easier phonation. As his voice began to respond, he found that the habitual extraneous movement of his head at vocal onset subsided. By the end of the session his voice was responding well. The following week, he reported less vocal strain during successive shows. However, he was still concerned about vocal strain. We shifted the focus to how he was standing and moving. During the show he not only sings but plays guitar and violin. The "Touch the Floor in Standing" lesson was used to help him find a better stance and flexibility for playing while moving around the stage. The importance of the lesson is learning to recognize holding patterns in the chest, neck, and shoulders. As we worked with this lesson, he noted changes in his ribs and shoulders as well as an increased sense of balance, because he was able to find ease of movement through his spine. He called after the next series of shows to report much more freedom of movement together with reduced vocal strain when performing.

Whether taught as a verbally directed *Awareness Through Movement* (ATM) lesson or a hands-on *Functional Integration* (FI) lesson, the Feldenkrais Method is a very important tool for somatic education for the professional voice user. Tension or discoordination, no matter how subtle, inhibits movement and can alter our desired vocal output.

Therefore, virtually any Feldenkrais lesson can have a positive impact on vocal quality and ease of phonation, since efficient vocal production cannot be separated from body mechanics. Which lessons have the most impact is totally dependent on the somatic needs of the specific student. A central feature of ATM lessons is the use of cues to draw the attention to various parts of the body. It is not necessary to add vocalization to a lesson, as the somatic changes during the lesson are often sufficiently powerful for the carryover to be automatic. However, it may be useful to repeat the basic movement of the lesson with vocalization to facilitate habituation of the pattern in another context.

References

Feldenkrais, M. (1949) 2005. *Body and Mature Behavior: A study of anxiety, sex, gravitation, and learning.* Reprint. Frog Books, Berkeley, CA.

Feldenkrais, M. 1995. *Dr. Moshe Feldenkrais at Alexander Yanai,* vols 1–12. International Feldenkrais Federation, Paris.

Giovanni, A., Akl, L., Ouaknine, M. 2008. Postural dynamics and vocal effort; preliminary experimental analysis. *Folia Phoniatrica et Logopedica* 60:80–85.

Kooijman, P., Dejong, F.I.C.R.S., Oudes, M.J., Huinck, W., Van Acht, H., Graamans, K. 2005. Muscular tension and body posture in relation to voice handicap and voice quality in teachers with persistent voice complaints. *Folia Phoniatrica et Logopedica* 57:134–147.

Lagier, A., Vaugoyeau, M., Ghio, A., Legou, T., Giovanni, A., Assaiante, C. 2010. Coordination between posture and phonation in vocal effort behavior. *Folia Phoniatrica et Logopedica* 62:195–202.

Lamperti, G.P. 2012. *The Technics of Bel Canto.* CreateSpace Independent Publishing Platform, Scotts Valley, CA.

LeBorgne, W., Rosenberg, M. 2014. *The Vocal Athlete.* Plural Publishing, San Diego, CA.

Lessac, A. 1997. *The Use and Training of the Human Voice,* 3rd edn. Mayfield Publishing, Mountain View, CA.

Nacci, A., Fattori, B., Mancini, V., Panicucci, E., Matteuccu, J., Ursino, S., Berrettini. S. 2012. Posturographic analysis in patients with dysfunctional dysphonia before and after speech therapy/rehabilitation treatment. *Acta Otophinolaryngologica Italica* 32:115–121.

Pettersen, V. 2005. Muscular patterns and activation levels of auxiliary muscles and thorax movement in classical singing. *Folia Phoniatrica et Logopedica* 57:255–277.

Questel, A., St. Cyr, T. 1995. "Interview of Alan Questel by Tommie St. Cyr," [Reprinted with permission from Association of Theatre Movement Educators (ATME) January 1995-Volume 3, Number 1] Available online at: https://www.feldenkraisguild.com/article_content.asp?edition=1&section=20&article=75. [Accessed October 13, 2020].

Rollins, E. 2017. The effects of heel height on head position, long-term average spectra, and perceptions of female singings. *Journal of Voice* 32(1):127.e15-127.e23. doi: 10.1016/j.jvoice.2017.03.005

Watson, A.H.D., Williams, C., James, B.V. 2012. Activity Patterns in latissimus dorsi and sternocleidomastoid in classical singers. *Journal of Voice* 26:95–105.

Equalizing the Nostrils *Awareness Through Movement* Audio Lesson taught by Marina Gilman

The dancer found her way onto her feet and then unfurled into an effortless arch backward. Her head leaned back as her abdomen released, allowing her ribs to open and her chest to float up. Her eyes widened as if entranced by a cosmic vision and "It's so ballet!" escaped her lips. She blossomed into a smile and let out a satisfied sigh as she was returning from her luxurious *cambré derrière*. This was just after an *Awareness Through Movement* (ATM) class I had taught at the Hong Kong Ballet before their daily company class.

This arching of the spine backward has been drilled and exercised time and time again in technique classes and in rehearsals, but, after the ATM, it was rather evoked. Without being told by anyone what she needed to do with her spine, or where her hips should be, or what her shoulder blades should be doing, the dancer knew exactly what needed to be done, because she was *feeling* herself. This *cambré derrière* is truly "so ballet" because it is a step often used in choreography to convey sweet euphoria or warm reverie. For this dancer, it became an integrated corporal expression that grew out of self-knowing and self-understanding, which had been brought about by a heightened state of self-listening instead of through strenuous work and forceful determination.

Watching her was so moving because she was unfolding into motion with another taste and appreciation – another layer of feeling – for who she was and what she was capable of. Her presence was more vibrant. This new sensation not only guided her to improve her dancing, but enabled her to savor an elevated refinement in her breathing, her stability, the turning of her head – her actions of living.

She could have stepped into the role of Juliet right then and there, breathing life into the choreography that expressed her innocent abandonment into the ecstasy of first-time love. She was living the moment. No longer trying but being. Being dance. Being living, moving art.

Now *this* is expression; this is artistic, I re-realized cheerfully inside myself. It was certainly not the first time I had seen a dancer awaken to the magic that they were, yet it continues to excite me to witness it happening again. Especially straight after an ATM lesson, there is a sensory buzz that's tangible throughout themselves, which informs finer articulation, curiosity, wonder, new understandings, and enjoyment as they test drive themselves through a movement exploration. They get carried into movement feeling either that their bodies know exactly what to do to meet the challenges of any ideas they propose to themselves, or that they are able to track every part of themselves to be more precise in finding ways to be on balance and smooth.

The studio began to fill up with the other dancers, signaling that it was time to get back to usual business. My student rolled up her yoga mat and went to her usual spot at the barre for the *plié* exercise. Her *pliés* were not so usual, however. They were imbued by something new she had learned – a deeper, embodied acquaintance with herself – that afforded her technical resilience to support the freedom of her creative and artistic fancy. She was approaching each exercise with more skill to negotiate a balance between the demands of the ballet language and her health, which empowered the spectacular expression of her own unique human potential.

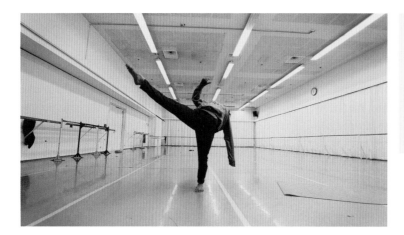

Figure 15.1
Sayaka Kado, a dancer with the Hessiches Staatsballett in Wiesbaden, finds her full range to extend backward after an ATM lesson with a book on the foot.

Courtesy of Paul Pui Wo Lee

Freedom from learning beyond schooling

I discovered Feldenkrais when I suffered two minor neck hernias back when I was dancing full-time at the contemporary dance company in Gothenburg.

"Between C4 and C5, and C6 and C7," I would recite to all the specialists. I was first referred to the best rehabilitation centre, and an hour-long program of strengthening exercises was designed for me. Although I did notice some improvements, I could still feel the presence of my neck injury. The image of wrapping layers of bandages over a leaky faucet kept popping up in my mind. Deep inside I didn't feel like the *real* problem was being addressed by a prescribed strengthening regime. My gut told me that I needed a way to discover how I could move *differently*, so I may dance with freedom and be protected at the same time.

I had always been very insecure as a dancer, but I was magnificent at masking the internal suspicion that I didn't actually know what I was doing. My encounter with the Feldenkrais Method confirmed that my suspicion was quite true. I felt that I didn't even know how to stand properly on my two feet. I was constantly analyzing other dancers and myself

even when just trying to hold a simple balance. I kept thinking that it surely can't be this mentally draining! The phenomenal dancers I admired all shared a quality of ease in everything they did, so I knew that I hadn't figured out the key to that yet. How could I move like liquid mercury – like a Cloud Gate dancer? How could my head draw freely through space like the Pina Bausch dancers? What is it about Forsythe dancers that they can move through extreme and contorted positions with agility and unconventional logic? How do Batsheva dancers, Rosas, Trisha…?

At my first *Functional Integration* (FI) lesson, after listening patiently to my lengthy outpouring about my injury, my Feldenkrais practitioner asked me to lie on my back. He quickly shared an observation:

"Your ribs don't move when you breathe."

"What ribs?"

My response revealed just what little concept I had of my ribs. Soon though, I heard a stream of voices from the past resurface. In no time, it was clear that my neck injury was no coincidence…

I had another rib-related epiphany a few months later during my first ATM class. We were lying on our backs, sliding one hand diagonally downward

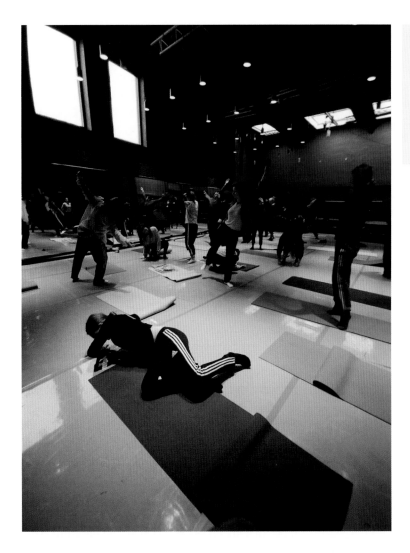

Figure 15.2
Dancers at Sceneindgangen in Copenhagen improvising with their new sensations after an *Awareness Through Movement* lesson.

Courtesy of Paul Pui Wo Lee

to reach away from the body and then returning. Such a simple movement, but it seemed impossible to me. It wasn't until the teacher suggested that I try allowing my head to roll and use the possibility of the ribs to fold on one side and open on the opposite side that my hand was actually going somewhere.

A light bulb didn't switch on – my mind exploded and lit up a galaxy! My rib cage can bend? I realized that I had been holding myself back all along.

Throughout my ballet education and my professional career, I didn't remember hearing much about my ribs other than that I should keep them down or "put them away." I got the idea that the rib cage was not something to be moved but fixed. I had also heard somewhere that belly breathing was better for the voice, which prompted me to move my ribs even less. I had subconsciously assimilated these ideas into my normal way of being.

The lesson proceeded to sliding and reaching my hand at different angles away from and toward my torso. It was so pleasurable to feel how my head could roll and how my chest could be more malleable to facilitate the movement of my arms, yet I could also notice that there was a programmed fear that it was somehow incorrect technique. When I stood up, to my surprise, I was naturally standing more solidly on my feet, yet I was more mobile than ever. My ribcage felt like it was this enormous fishing net in the ocean that billowed in different directions. I was moving through the studio feeling such fullness and range in my every move. Everything felt connected and I barely needed to think and piece each step together separately. I was listening to my body and my body was listening to me. My arms would smoothly follow whatever my torso would propose. This classic correction in dancing of "the arms come from your back" finally had meaning in my body – in myself. I doubt that any amount of words or industrious hard work would have gotten me to that quality of embodied understanding. I was practically screaming inside, "Why did I not get this at school? Why didn't I know about this Feldenkrais earlier!?"

This was how I had been wanting to dance all these years. I finally felt like I was an honest modern dancer who could enjoy doing a Limón class and be high with the thrill of truly knowing how to move and fulfill the spirit of that style rather than just replicating the form. I continued to let my amazement and self-discoveries unfold in the studio with this new feeling of myself. My head was swaying freely, my ribs bending and opening easily, and my spine yielded to entertain the whims of my improvised movement exploration. I somehow got the message that I didn't need to rely on just my neck to move my head. I had my entire self to help me, and my neck injury began fading into the background.

Learning to dance does not equal learning optimal self-use

Learning to dance can be seen in the same way as learning to write. You start with the basics, which would be the letters of the alphabet. Once you can form these, you advance to putting the letters together to form words; words link up to become phrases; phrases turn into sentences; sentences into paragraphs; and these accumulate into essays, novels, etc. I always say that Feldenkrais is that which helps you learn and refine the way you do that essential thing so obvious that it can be forgotten – how to hold the pen. Dancers learn to dance, but they do not necessarily invest in learning how to move with more intelligence, sensitivity, and wisdom, allowing them to convert their intentions into action efficiently. Often, the mentality is simply to push harder to overcome challenges.

I consider the benefits of injury prevention and recovery that are engrained in the spirit of Feldenkrais as being a method of artistic deepening. Through getting to know our human material, we reduce the unnecessary and extraneous strain that causes damage and hampers our improvement, so that we may expand the ways in which we can mobilize our human design with a higher degree of collaboration, and uncover sounder and more sustainable ways to move that are no less spectacular and beautiful. This learning about our potential improves our craft by offering us the opportunity to peek into new possibilities of creating art that simultaneously rejuvenate the vibrancy of the material from which we derive our art.

There are very few dancers who can lift their legs and their hands properly because they are instructed how to do it. And you have learned it from somebody else.

Feldenkrais 1981

Dancing entails moving in a stylized way, and dancers are schooled to move according to a certain

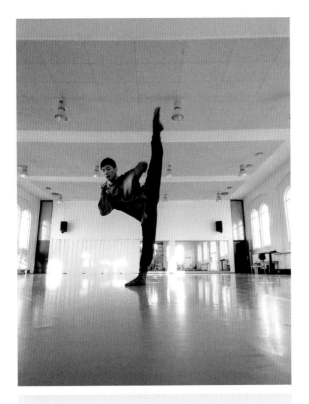

Figure 15.3
I was 'Mr. 45-degrees' back in ballet school. Feldenkrais helped me discover flexibility beyond (what we hold to be) the rules.

Courtesy of Paul Pui Wo Lee

aesthetic standard or code. These notions of right and wrong adopted from external sources – their teachers, coaches, and what they observe in the works of choreographers – are indeed useful and fundamental to train them for a basic level of proficiency in the style of dance they have chosen. However, the abidance by these "rules" can be the very hindrance to their competence and progress, and the rules they move by are sometimes re-evaluated only after injury.

I was rather shocked at how dancers would hurt themselves doing the gentlest and simplest movements in my ATM classes. Some would endure the pain from the position instructed or from the movements, and it became increasingly clear how dancers can favor the rules and beliefs they've acquired over listening to their own signals of pain and discomfort.

Some dancers do sense that what they are doing in their dancing causes them discomfort but cannot yet imagine other ways of moving that will help them improve. Feldenkrais offers a situation outside their usual pressure of the aesthetic standard, so they may explore and come across new ways of moving their skeleton that might otherwise be unavailable to them in their usual dance context.

Teaching versus creating the conditions for knowledge to be understood

External guidance and feedback from teachers is tremendously useful. However, the majority of corrections are communicated through demonstration and words, and because their interpretation varies from person to person, this can lead eventually to different movement inefficiencies. For example, to improve the backbend, you might be told to open your chest, think about lifting from your sternum, pull your shoulders back, lengthen your front, use your back, or other similar instructions. The language used in dance instruction doesn't encompass the complexity and accuracy of the anatomical happenings that constitute the steps. Improved precision in how a person approaches the unveiling of solutions to technical or artistic issues is nevertheless possible.

Where does the back actually arch from? Does it happen in a portion of the spine where only a few vertebrae are involved? Would that be more in the upper back or lower back? Or is arching happening as an event involving the whole spine? Is the pelvis a factor, and could it be a contributing element? How does the sternum fit in? What is the role of the muscles of the lower belly, and how does that relate to the availability of the lumbar vertebrae? If there was a manual written that included all the fine details of the functional movement connections of our anatomy during the backbend, would studying that manual provide more practical knowledge toward doing the step successfully?

What I am trying to get at is that there is another way of communicating through a different language, one that is common to all people: sensation. What if, instead of saying, "I will tell you what needs to happen," we offer, "May I help you sense what it feels like for all those things to happen?" Going down to the floor and experiencing small bits of the necessary movements and connections within the skeleton can give a corporal, comprehensive understanding of what was intended behind the words in a more immediate way.

This is why I decided to teach the ATM called "Making the Sternum Flexible" at the Hong Kong Ballet. I see the lesson as helping dancers recognize the colors on their palette more clearly, so they can

have a broader overview of what is available to aid their discovery of more combined expressive possibilities. Can you use what you can't see or perceive fully? Dancers are artists, and therefore naturally wish to excel. Like their nervous system, they do the best with what they know, so allowing them to *sense* the individual human material at their disposal (i.e., themselves), they are provided with more detailed information to be resourceful. Through sensing, they can apply themselves toward their artistic visions and ambitions in ways that honor their *individual* potential as artists and human beings.

Feldenkrais and ballet

The more Feldenkrais lessons I did, the more I felt *myself*, and surprisingly enough I would look more "classical" in ballet class. Not only was I twisting, arching, and bending in adherence to the classical aesthetic, but there was a functional logic to the shapes I was passing through. After many ATMs, I would experience a high-definition quality sensation of myself that opened me up to go into a movement flow with curiosity. I found that I could mold

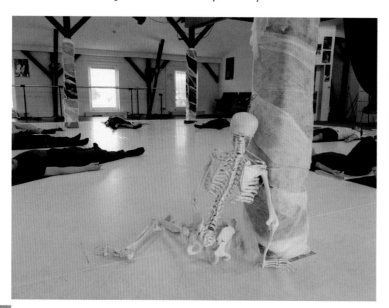

Figure 15.4
Artistic revolution – incorporating Feldenkrais as a part of the company warm-up class at Of Curious Nature, a contemporary dance company in Bremen.

Courtesy of Paul Pui Wo Lee

this groove, or mode of moving, according to the parameters of ballet. I was much more technically secure than when I tried hard, and I had more liberty in my expressive decisions. I was eager to share this with other dancers, since I knew that many struggled with this seemingly rigid and challenging style, even though it's still a common warm-up before rehearsals.

What I observe the moment after an ATM lesson is what could be called a cycle of self-inspiration. Most dancers will immerse themselves in their own bath of sensory input and enter a continuum of movement exploration and research. It is a potent state where dancers see themselves sharply through movement and can continue to feel how the learning from the ATM spills into and informs their usual way of moving. Sometimes the dancers follow the pull of their sensations; sometimes they intentionally challenge the organizational ability of their nervous system and experience it recover their balance.

Moving into the ballet class, I remind the dancers to take it as structured improvisation. Almost everyone knows ballet language and protocol, so I encourage them to be bold in allowing themselves to follow their sensations within the framework of the ballet vocabulary and trust that their acquired "knowing" of themselves will bring sensibility, creativity, and technical assurance to shape their flow through the classical forms.

The exercises I give are only propositions and serve only as a guideline for dancers to play with. I want them to experience how their enhanced sensation of themselves is organizing them toward more sustainable and wholesome patterns of moving that could lead to unimagined expressive and technical feats. I hope to help them cultivate the seemingly lost art of enjoying dance and to trust that by meeting each step with fascination for their own potential they will form their own poetry in motion.

I understand Feldenkrais to be a method that empowers the dignity of the artist. It equips the dancer to have the maturity to seek answers from themself and to continue developing beyond what their teachers wished to convey. I hope it will be cherished in the dancer's toolbox as a means of expanding and optimizing the use of their artistic material – their living – to enrich both their craft and their quality of being human.

References

Feldenkrais, M. 1981. *Amherst Training Transcriptions*, June 9. International Feldenkrais Federation, Paris.

Other resources

[All videos accessed October 2020]

Alon, R. "Movement Nature Meant Part I" https://youtu.be/igpJeOkgfzw

Batsheva Dance Company. Ohad Naharin,"Three" https://youtu.be/rCaHbOLGXfY

Bausch, P. "Vollmond" https://youtu.be/u15d-AT9OLg

Bausch, P. "Vollmond Arte 2013 06 26" https://youtu.be/m4d-mHjtCG8

Cloud Gate Dance Theatre. "Cursive II" https://youtu.be/nGQIrTs2FAw "Moon Water" https://youtu.be/KmTplJXenAg

De Keersmaeker, A.T. "Achterland" https://youtu.be/mTCIVAXDstk Rosas/"Drumming" https://youtu.be/vZEcwHBBQhI

Forsythe, W. "Solo" https://www.youtube.com/watch?v=hDTu7jF_EwY "One Flat Thing, reproduced" https://youtu.be/SGvfqpQZC-s

Paxton, S. "Material for the Spine" https://youtu.be/8CntWmA1YTw

Wenders, W. "Pina," Trailer for documentary about Pina Bausch https://www.youtube.com/watch?v=LHJH9-r6xp0

Making the Sternum More Flexible *Awareness Through Movement* Audio Lesson taught by Paul Pui Wo Lee

Introduction: a theatrically cultured man

This chapter discusses the application of the Feldenkrais Method as an enactivist, transformative process within theater-training and performance-making contexts.[1] It takes into account contemporary reflections on somatic-informed performance practices and developments in the field of theater and cognition, and gives insight into an emerging working practice with professional and student actors. There has been an increase in literature on the Feldenkrais Method as a resource for actors' training and practice, highlighting issues concerning performer-agency, skills acquisition, and holistic communication. This is part of a trend in Western actor training that embraces 20th-century somatic practices as a resource for a holistic education. Such a trend recognizes movement as a fundamental agency-constituting experience and parallels scholarly developments in actor training and theater reception that draws on studies in cognitive sciences concerned with notions of autonomy, embodiment, kinesthetic empathy, imagination, and affect (Blair and Cook 2016).

Moshe Feldenkrais developed a playful practice of self-education and "awarded learning" that aims to empower learners through fostering an "understanding of the somatic aspects of consciousness" (Feldenkrais 2010, p. 34). He aimed to facilitate conditions in which learners could develop flexible minds through creative and attentive interaction with the world. It is this flexibility, being

"amendable to change" (2010, p. xvii), which is also at the heart of Western theater practice. Actors need to be able to incorporate and adapt to different roles and situations with ease, curiosity, nuanced control, and imagination as part of their daily work context. Contemporary neuroplasticity researchers suggest that learning modalities within the Feldenkrais Method foster brain plasticity. Michael Merzenich argues that "our brain is continuously changing by what we do. And what we do really matters, because what we do represents the basis for the creation of the person who we are" (Merzenich and Baniel 2013). This *doing* as the "basis for the creation of the person who we are," is at the heart of the principles found in the actor training systems based on the work of Konstantin Stanislavski (1863–1938) and his disciples, who developed processes of *Actioning* as toolkits for character development and scene work (Merzenich and Baniel 2013). Stanislaviski's exercises were based not upon emotion, as is sometimes thought, but upon action. Emotion, he thought, arises properly from the action, not the reverse (Turner 1963, p. 320).

Feldenkrais was familiar with the post-Stanislavski acting systems developed in Russia, Israel, and the US. He suggested that an actor needed to be trained "to have the fluent ability to act and check what his actions mean in reality" (Feldenkrais and Schechner 1966, p. 118). This awareness of action fosters capacity to properly listen and respond to another actor on the stage and allows the assumption of the characteristics required for a role to happen with "greater clarity and ease" (p. 125), while also rediscovering their body's capability and potential (Feldenkrais and Schechner 1966, p. 123).

---

1 Enactivism, an evolving field within cognitive sciences, can provide a theoretical framework echoing constructivist ideas and methods put forward by Feldenkrais. It proposes cognition as grounded in the dynamics of the sensorimotor interactions between the living organism and its environment (Steward et al. 2014).

Feldenkrais' work is "concerned with learning a better mode of action and uses of the body, from which the person can learn directly, in his own body language" (cited in Reese 1985, p. 153). This ability is equally articulated in writings by Stanislavski, concerned with "organismic functioning of man," where thinking and feeling are necessarily an embodied whole (Prokofiev 1964, cited in Litvinoff 1972). Like Feldenkrais, he aimed to access the person's agency, creativity, and potential through movement.

We are more at home with physical action than with the elusive nature of emotion. Here we can find our bearing better, here we are more inventive, and more certain than with subjective elements which are difficult to capture and fix.

Prokofiev 1964, cited in Litvinoff 1972

Strange variations: awareness and creativity

Moshe Feldenkrais developed his practices as an ongoing process of embodied questioning of habitual modes of thought-patterning, self-perception, and world-perceiving. At the heart of his practice is a facilitating of conditions for the creative probing of variations and opposing solutions to given tasks or situations. Having access to a nuanced and open-ended process of embodied questioning forms an essential toolkit for the actor, within the processes of character development or scenic work. Recent literature on actor training highlights the importance of being accomplished in working through discovery-based processes. As Ewan and Green (2015, p. 6) propose, for the actor the interrogation and practice of movement is "a life-long commitment, a deepening process of discovery. Awareness of our moving self operates on many levels and so it is important for the actor to explore each level thoroughly."

In the Feldenkrais Method, learning is facilitated through *induction* (Feldenkrais 2010, p. 42) – emergent processes of knowledge creation through observation, discovery, and trial and error. Theater director Julia Pascal (interview with author, 2010) described the effect of Feldenkrais lessons as preparatory practices within professional rehearsal contexts:

The performers are examining sensation, using emotional and intellectual parts of the self at the same time; what you are doing is to encourage that flow,

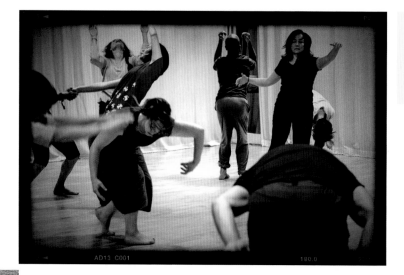

Figure 16.1
Rehearsal photo from the production of *The Dybbuk.*

Courtesy of Habie Schwarz

which the performers then take into rehearsal and into their performance. And that's the strongest effect I have ever seen in rehearsal – which is fantastic.

Actor Simeon Perlin (interview with author, August 8, 2010) describes the learning as offered through the Feldenkrais Method as "being encouraged to discover something in myself." Such encouragement toward self-discovery can foster greater creative risk-taking and learning for the actor. The capacity for transformation, and the ability to naturalize unfamiliar behavior patterns is a part of the actor's job. Pascal elaborates on the effects of a Feldenkrais-informed explorative rehearsal ethos toward accessing the performer's emerging potential:

You make the person experience their own bodies as if it's a new coat, and that is very exciting, and makes the person realize that they can expand and grow in a way they had not thought of before... That questioning which transmutes into a body change allows the person to widen and realize they are capable of much more.

interview with author, August 8, 2010

Psychiatrist Norman Doidge (2015) suggests that with Feldenkrais lessons the slowing down in execution of actions, the lowering of stimuli and muscle tonus, and the focus on the breaking down of larger patterns form powerful awareness-forming conditions. Actor Juliet Dante described the effect of Feldenkrais lessons as processes of "centring, opening, and focusing" (interview with author, August 8, 2010) – all useful as somatic tuning processes for the actor:

The movements are so gentle, and bring you back into yourself, but not only into yourself, it makes you aware of first of all your center – and then you open out; and everything is quite gentle, so it's very specific; no movement is gratuitous. So it helps to focus.

interview with author, August 8, 2010

Actor Stefan Karsberg identifies a link between an improved awareness and a potential for increased agility for the actor through Feldenkrais processes: "You become aware of parts of your body moving, particularly the feeling or the sensations of it... You are more active; a performer should be active at all points" (quoted in Kampe 2016). These actors' findings correlate with Feldenkrais' concept of *acture* (Feldenkrais 2005, p. 207): the ability of the learner to engage creatively with any situation under any given circumstances.

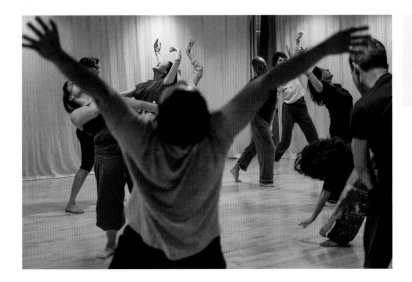

Figure 16.2
Rehearsal photo from the production of *The Dybbuk*.

Courtesy of Habie Schwarz

Enacting empathy

Empathy is at the heart of theatre, performance, and education. In order to connect with what the other person is feeling, we need empathy. The body – embodiment – remains central in current definitions of empathy in cognitive sciences. The science provides evidence for what teachers and theatre practitioners have felt intuitively is true – we are whole/holistic beings.

Blair 2015

Feldenkrais lessons offer non-corrective, pleasurable, and structured dialogues between practitioner and learner. These revolve around feedback-loops of mutual body-listening and adaption to new behavior, forming an empathetic social process which fosters brain plasticity.

Norman Doidge describes neurochemical processes of *globalization* in which conditions within the brain are created that influence "the overall effectiveness of the synaptic connections and bring about enduring change" in self-organization (Doidge 2007, p. 118). Doidge and other neuroscientists suggest that neuroplasticity – Feldenkrais' aim for "flexible minds" – and openness for change in behavior depend largely on a "fertilization" (Hüther 2012) of newly wired synaptic patterns and neuromodulators through our affective perception of pleasure, passion, and compassionate love. A key role of the Feldenkrais practitioner is to fertilize conditions for learning, discovery, and absorption of new behavior for the individual and between participants. Such fertilization acknowledges feeling and affect – pleasure, curiosity, fear, pain, and desire – in the relational process of learning, rehearsal, or performance making. Merzenich (2012) suggests that notions of motivation and inclusion of learner awareness in the witnessing of embodied learning processes are key Feldenkrais strategies that are both crucial for transformative learning and aligned with current research in brain plasticity rehabilitation. The Feldenkrais Method facilitates embodied conditions of self-witnessing through self-questioning. The questions asked, verbally or through touch, are concerned with linking a relational intentionality, agency, and pattern-recognition through movement. My performance pedagogy enhances such enacted questioning through a fertilizing (Hüther 2012) of such conditions, by providing a fluid layer of conditions for play and compassion.

"A completely different sense of self"

For the last 20 years I have worked with Feldenkrais-informed pedagogies as a teacher, artist, and researcher. The performance-making processes which I have explored in professional contexts have been reviewed as a transformative modality where the actors work "with all the power of bodily experience" (Merle Molofsky review of *The Dybbuk*, 2010 blog post, quoted in Kampe 2016). Students of the BA Acting programme at Bath Spa University (UK), where my Feldenkrais-informed movement pedagogies are integrated within a creative curriculum, have commented on changes in their ability to access reflective embodiment as a fundamental modality for learning and creative practice. Students articulated their growing ability to link embodiment and action to sensing, feeling, and thinking. Such awareness and curiosity toward accessing this affective/cognitive unity through movement has inspired students to explore creative choices as actors. Year 1 student Matt reflects:

I feel much more confident and defined within my movement, believing that I can now tell a story/narrative through expressing my body and emotions, accessing a vast amount of different movements whilst playing with tempo and rhythm. I now feel I have the ability to link my inner attitudes to the actions and intentions that I play as an actor on stage and in the moment. I feel my link to breath and inner attitude is now embodied throughout my work and displays clarity and precision.

Fellow student Alex expands on a Feldenkrais-informed competence in embodied acting, which

has transferred especially well into text work, allowing me to find a matching physical and vocal expression when performing. This has helped me establish the psycho-physical bond we learn about in Stanislavski's work, making my performances as an actor much more embodied.

Students are experiencing a syllabus that encourages them to retranslate their bodily experience into verbal language, and where practical learning is framed through contextual reading about Feldenkrais and other somatic modalities. During their first semester of study, students begin to develop their own practice by using fragments of ATM lessons as a daily preparatory process to construct ease, flexibility, readiness, and agility. Asking students to work in self-directed ways toward inhabiting and enacting their own gentle tuning processes is an important step toward learner autonomy. Student Billie-Jo reflects on developing her own self-directed tuning practice, as well as on transferring Feldenkrais processes experienced over the first year of study outside the classroom situation:

I now do a small daily warm up, so that I am up and ready for the day and am more aware of tension and aches in my body than I was before. In other (Feldenkrais) classes I think about my body in space and how by using physical actions I can evoke emotions instead of just using words.

The importance of pleasure and comfort as a point of departure for affective communication was also highlighted by students:

I am far more comfortable now in my own body. My flexibility has improved vastly and I am more

coordinated. I feel more confident to express my emotion through movement. I feel I am able to communicate more clearly.

Chloe, Year 1 in 2013

Students suggested that a shift in self-perception toward being more grounded, centered, and open toward their spatial and social environment created an improved competence and confidence toward creative practice. Student Larnaca in 2019 describes herself as:

… a lot more grounded, as if I have more of a relationship with the floor and an awareness of the space around me. I am able to feel taller, which gives me more authority on stage. I now understand the importance of being able to react and move on impulse, particularly through touch of the other people I am working with. This helps with truth and authenticity.

There are several problems and limitations when applying the Feldenkrais Method in performer training or artistic contexts. Time constraints in classroom situations and the need to achieve distinct results, learning outcomes, or artistic products are cultural conditions which can conflict with Feldenkrais' strategies of induction, the absence of demonstration in ATM lessons and its non-corrective stance toward learner agency and progress. Furthermore, Feldenkrais lessons can seem dynamically and spatially limited in artistic contexts, owing to the method being sensory based and introspective rather than immediately affective, spatially expansive, and dynamically expressive.

My teaching draws on Feldenkrais lessons, strategies and principles, but also utilizes Rudolf Laban's dynamic and spatial studies to enhance qualitative variations of affective experience of the learner within embodied interactions with the world, and to stimulate "a learning process that makes

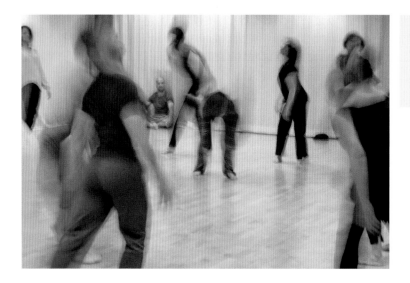

Figure 16.3
Rehearsal photo from the production of *The Dybbuk.*

Courtesy of Habie Schwarz

self-direction easier and more pleasurable" (Feldenkrais 2010, p. 67). It also extends Feldenkrais' *Functional Integration* touch-based dialogues into partner-interaction principles emerging from Contact Improvisation and basic acrobatic practices. Such touch-based practices seem appropriate to support the transformational processes of Feldenkrais' learning modalities that aim to view the learner as a reflective, dynamic, and desiring social creature. Student Matt (2018) comments on his growing competence in using movement and touch as relational rehearsal tools, where he is able to "use touch during rehearsals to bring a new dynamic to a scene, and movement explorations to bring new life and spontaneity to a piece."

My teaching of Movement for Actors acknowledges the transformative and agency-forming potential of a somatic-informed pedagogy. I weave Feldenkrais' dignified humanist ethos and organic principles into the overarching fabric of my pedagogy. This includes teaching through questioning, slowing down to give time for self- and peer-observation through action/reflection cycles, and a facilitating of conditions for learning through small approximations. Through the use of repetition, variation, defamiliarization, and disorientation, I aim to construct a dialogue between familiarity and a provocative "novelty of situation" (Feldenkrais 2010, p. 37). While creating a nonnormative environment for pleasurable enquiry, I encourage students to test and extend their limitations in their actions and self-image in non-threatening ways through improvisational explorations. This allows learners to experience heightened force, speed, precision, and a sense of abandon and expansiveness, and to transfer their newly acquired self-image into creative situations that anticipate the often highly dynamic demands of theatrical practice.

As a pedagogue, I consistently need to balance a non-corrective learner-centered stance that supports the development of an autonomous person through movement, and a goal-oriented mode of skills development training that meets professional demands. Year Two student Iulian (2013) describes the dialogue between a pleasurable change in self-perception and an increase in embodied professional competence:

It gave me confidence and purpose in movement, and it opened a new world for me, widening my movement palette. It made me feel great, more aware of what my body is saying and being braver in movement. It changed my perception of relating through movement completely from the point of view of energy, force, and meaning, making me more confident and open about movements that I never even dreamt I could ever do.

Conclusion

My Feldenkrais-informed pedagogy of Movement for Actors aims to enhance students' ability to access embodiment and experience as tools for organic and transformative learning. It further aims to facilitate performer agency by enabling students to embrace an embodied relational sense of self as a flexible resource for creative inquiry. Students develop high levels of competence as moving actors, and learn to work in safe, constructive, and sustainable ways in professional contexts. Year 1 student Morgan (2019) reflects on a change toward a growing autonomy in self-image, learning, and artistic choice-making through movement at the end of her first year at university:

I used to judge myself very harshly when it came to movement, as I felt there was not a lot I could do. However, I feel that I have improved a lot and this has helped me to judge myself less and stop me from comparing myself to others. I am much more comfortable in using my body to express myself than I was at the start of the year, and this enables me to fully embody what I am trying to say and make my feelings clear. I also now think about how I am moving as a character that I need to take on, and how I can fully embody the role. My sense of alignment and posture have improved since the beginning of the year and I am able to find my neutral alignment with ease. I am much more active in general and I

now have a desire to exercise more frequently, as it improves my self-esteem.

In this chapter I have placed the Feldenkrais Method as an enactivist model of somatic education into the context of neuroplasticity research and theater practice, which offers a rich and tangible praxis that can serve as a resource for transformative arts learning. I suggest that the transfer of Feldenkrais practices into more dynamically varied improvisational explorations might enhance affective neuro-flexibility in the learner and create greater potential for autonomy in making choices. I have described an embodied process of self-creation that redistributes touch-interaction within the Feldenkrais Method beyond the hierarchical limitations of a dialogue between practitioner and learner. Touch-based practice transforms the learning of acting into a process of learning through interaction and enaction – a shared becoming. Such pedagogy deserves further attention toward the facilitation of self-directed and co-creative learning. Bath Spa University's BA Acting students awarded the Feldenkrais-informed pedagogy they had experienced in their studies as "The Most Innovative Teaching" in 2015, suggesting that it helped them to free their creativity, build their confidence, and enjoy what they were doing. Students described how such an educational experience invoked spiritual, political, emotional, and physical realizations that brightened and enriched their lives.

References

Blair, R. 2015. Notes on Empathy, Cognitive Neuroscience, and Theatre/Education. *p-e-r-f-o-r-m-a-n-c-e* 2(1–2). http://p-e-r-f-o-r-m-a-n-c-e.org/?p=1101

Blair, R., Cook, A. 2016. *Theatre, Performance and Cognition: Languages, bodies and ecologies.* Bloomsbury, London.

Doidge, N. 2007. *The Brain that Changes Itself: Stories of personal triumph from the frontiers of brain science.* Penguin, New York, NY.

Doidge, N. 2015. *The Brain's Way of Healing: Remarkable discoveries and recoveries from the frontiers of neuroplasticity.* Scribe Publications, London.

Ewan, V., Green, D. 2015. *Actor Movement: Expression of the physical being.* Bloomsbury, London.

Feldenkrais, M. 2005. *Body and Mature Behaviour: A study of anxiety, sex, gravitation and learning,* 2nd edn. International Universities Press, Madison, WI.

Feldenkrais, M. 2010. In: E. Beringer (ed.) *Embodied Wisdom: The collected papers of Moshe Feldenkrais.* North Atlantic Books, Berkeley, CA.

Feldenkrais, M., Schechner, R. 1966. *Image, Movement, and Actor: Restoration of potentiality,* translated and edited by Kelly Morris. http://www.feldenkraismethod. com/wp-content/uploads/2014/11/Image-Movement-and-Actor-Moshe-Feldenkrais.pdf

Hüther, G. 2012. *Was wir sind und was wir sein könnten.* Fischer, Frankfurt.

Kampe, T. 2016. "crossing/weaving": somatic interventions in choreographic practices. *Feldenkrais Research Journal* 5:19. Available online at: http:// iffresearchjournal.org/system/files/FRJ-5-Kampe-161129.pdf

Litvinoff, V. 1972. *The Use of Stanislavski Within Modern Dance.* American Dance Guild Inc., New York, NY.

Merzenich, M. 2012. "Dr. Michael Merzenich on Neuroscience, Learning and the Feldenkrais Method." https:// www.youtube.com/watch?v=rupZ-wlRdA0

Merzenich, M., Baniel, A. 2013. "Brain Plasticity and Transformation." Video clip of conversation. https://www. youtube.com/watch?v=Jf_08J2Ete4

Reese, M. 1985. "Moshe Feldenkrais' work with movement: A parallel approach to Milton Erickson's hypnotherapy." *Ericksonian Psychotherapy, Vol. 1.* Brunner and Mazel, New York, NY.

Steward, J., Gapenne, O., Di Paolo, E.A. 2014. *Enaction: Towards a new paradigm for cognitive science.* MIT Press, Cambridge, MA.

Turner, W.L. 1963. Vakhtangov: The director as teacher. *Educational Theatre Journal* 15(4):318–326

Other resources

Doidge, N. 2015. "Interview about the Feldenkrais Method." https://www.youtube.com/watch?v=eKNBYzoOICQ

Feldenkrais, M. 1952. *Higher Judo: Groundwork.* Frederick Warne, London.

Kampe, T. 2015. Eros and Inquiry: The Feldenkrais Method as a complex process. *Theatre, Dance and Performance Training* 6(2):200–212. https://www.tandfonline.com/doi/ full/10.1080/19443927.2015.1027451

Worsley, V. 2016. *Feldenkrais for Actors: How to do less and discover more.* Nick Hern Books, London.

Worsley, V. 2019. "From the Coal Face": Teaching Feldenkrais on UK vocational drama trainings. *Feldenkrais Research Journal* 6. https://feldenkraisresearchjournal. org/index.php/journal/article/view/14

I first discovered the Feldenkrais Method in 1991 when I was playing rugby internationally and recovering from a series of concussions. I found it so quickly effective in my own healing process, and congruent with my professional and academic training in Sport and Exercise Science and Biomechanics, that I decided to enroll in a professional training program. I have now been practicing the method for 28 years.

Through my various experiences as an athletic trainer, a sports and conditioning specialist, and a Feldenkrais practitioner, I have worked with many athletes from the recreational level to the elite.

Learning skill, not will

Learning, as I see it, is not the training of willpower but the acquisition of the skill to inhibit parasitic action and the ability to direct clear motivations as a result of self-knowledge.

Feldenkrais 1985, Introduction

Adam Oates is a National Hockey League Hall of Fame player and former head coach of the Washington Capitals. Later, he set up the Oates Sports Group and now spends his time as a private hockey coach, working with NHL players to develop their craft on the ice.

We met at a golf resort where I was teaching Feldenkrais to golfers, and started talking. He told me that, during his 19 years as a professional player and coach (and then, in his retirement, as a pretty good golfer), he had traveled around North America and met with many of the top strength and conditioning specialists, but not one of them had been able to address fundamental questions about how their strength-training methods transferred to an improvement in the rotational aspects of their golf swing, or helped any one of their hockey players skate, turn, and shoot the puck in a high-speed, collision-heavy environment. I gave him a lesson and after that, he started to attend my classes.

In Adam's first individual Feldenkrais lesson with me, it was quickly revealed how unprepared he was to shift his weight onto his right leg and turn, owing to a former knee injury and lack of proprioceptive and spatial awareness on that side. This improved quickly during our lessons, and when he realized Feldenkrais' value and superiority over the vast array of training modalities to which he had been exposed in earlier years, he was drawn to study the method in greater depth.

Over the last ten years, together we have developed some new ways of incorporating the Feldenkrais Method into hockey players' training routines as a way to assist in their recovery, rehabilitate from injuries, acquire skills, and enhance their performance.

Developing core ability and agility

Precise and coordinated body motion is critical to achievement in competitive sports. Proprioception, or kinesthesia, is "the perception of the motion of the joint and body, and the position of the body or body segments in space." In movement science research, there is increasing knowledge of the role that sensory data plays in neuroplasticity. The brain incorporates and integrates proprioceptive data from a multitude of joint and muscle receptors, and interoceptors to regulate and refine motion patterns.

Spontaneity is a subjective and relative notion... It depends on the internal sensation of resistance experienced while acting or inhibiting action.

Feldenkrais 1985, p. 6

Athletic skills require agility and coordination, the major ingredients of functional strength. Many athletes who want to enhance their power exercise to improve their strength, rather than practicing activities to improve their agility, dexterity, and coordination.

If you only train toward strength without agility and coordination, it is, over time, destructive to the joints and the connective tissue of the human body. Without agility and coordination, without movement efficiency, our muscles only contract when we are tense – this exaggerates already-existing imbalances that create damaging, shearing forces across joints.

Some of the basic principles of the Feldenkrais Method that are related to my way of working with athletes are:

- **Proportional distribution of muscular effort:** The big muscles do the big work and the small muscles do the small work.

- **The skeleton** affords ideal paths of action.

- **Force must travel through the joints,** not across or around them, in order to avoid shearing forces. Soft tissue is available for action, but is ineffective for support.

- **Evenly distributed muscular tone:** No place works harder than any other place. A well-organized person experiences lightness and ease in movement.

- **Balance/counterbalance:** Improved balance is achieved when the center of the body mass is clearly organized above the base of support.

- **Orientation is a biological necessity** and is essential to all action. Spatial relationships and coordination are determined by orientation.

- **Every action** has the components of manipulation, orientation, and timing/coordination.

I use Feldenkrais as a way of developing true functional strength, so that athletes can perform an action with a clear "felt sense" of their intention in relation to the goals they want to achieve.

There is a functional interdependence between the musculoskeletal and central nervous systems. In this sensorimotor loop, changes that occur in one part of the system will be reflected by adaptations elsewhere within the system. Neurologically, neurons that fire together, wire together. In a way, every motor skill is a circuit, and through correct technique and practice, each skill is formed and optimized. Precision practice is informed and aided by clear proprioceptive feedback which, in turn, creates new myelination of the circuit. These new synaptic connections, like high-speed/capacity bandwidth, create a highly adaptable brain and nervous system that is better able to predict and respond appropriately to the quickly changing environment in competition.

In the process of *Functional Integration* movement sessions, new coordinative synergies are created that improve movement efficiency and reduce internal muscular resistance to action. Fluidity and spontaneity in action are experienced and learned through varied repetition.

What is useful for my students is this felt sense of movement efficiency: of being able to perform the same amount of work with a lot less effort. Athletes, with their high kinesthetic acuity, learn this distinction quickly. They specifically learn to let their antigravity reflexes work for them, creating dynamic equilibrium. As they discover this new

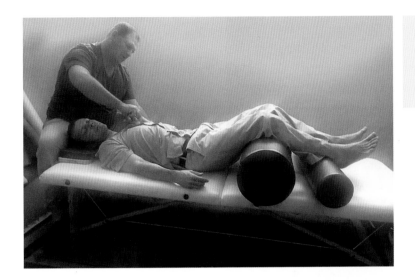

Figure 17.1
Dwight Pargee giving a
Functional Integration lesson.

Courtesy of Dwight Pargee

type of stability and agility of "central control" of their tonic musculature, they have more ease of movement and less compression through the whole musculoskeletal system. They learn to use awareness – embodied awareness, spatial awareness, and movement awareness – so that their long-held patterns of movement, posture, breathing, and muscular tension are changed. It is a wonderful experience to feel how your brain reorganizes itself at the neuromuscular level, and appreciate how this affects movement timing, coordination, power, and speed.

Our human evolutionary biology is predicated upon the idea of adaptability, resiliency, mobility, and movement. When an athlete is injured, their neuromuscular system develops a protection strategy to prevent further damage occurring, by reducing the degrees of freedom and movement variability. For example, when someone sprains their ankle, their motor control becomes impaired, so they will feel unstable when they are standing on the injured leg. This protective strategy is global; it shows up in the pelvic musculature and in the antigravity musculature of the spine, as well as in the

head and neck relationship. As a defense mechanism, it is a biologically intelligent response to the trauma at the time of the injury, because the brain is trying to prevent more damage from occurring.

As humans, we have the biological capacity to observe what we are doing and refine our action in the world. In the Feldenkrais Method, we refer to this as *Awareness*, with a big A. We can change our self-image, the neurological body maps which inform our thinking, sensing, emotional feeling, and acting/moving in the world. All these are happening simultaneously; and this unity of self and our environment is constant and immutable. Our behaviors have to do with our responses to the current situation, along with all of our own personal history.

Case Study: the story of JP

At the time of writing, JP is a star player and veteran leader of his NHL team. He is known for his strength, athleticism, and speed on the ice, and has

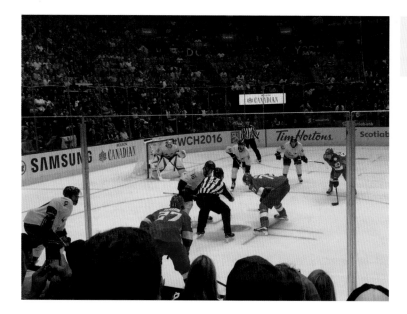

Figure 17.2

Courtesy of Staffan Elgelid

been a prolific scorer throughout his professional career. His high work rate around the net and bulldog-like approach to winning the puck was a successful playing strategy early on in his career. In his early 30s, after several injury-plagued years, he began to realize that he needed to develop another skillset to prolong his career.

I saw him after the end of a season. As I was interviewing him, he revealed that he had suffered a couple of concussions early in the season that had set him back. He stated that he wanted to be able to turn to the right more quickly and felt that his neck and shoulders were stiff, limiting his turning ability. He had also realized through feedback with Coach Oates that his current approach to winning the puck at any cost put him down on the ice too much and set him up for more injury opportunities. He felt he needed to be able to lean back into his stance while maintaining balance on his feet, and improve his peripheral vision in order to better see players and puck movement and therefore better anticipate where to position himself more effectively.

As I assessed his standing balance and turning ability over each leg, it became immediately obvious that he was guarding his right hip joint; he was not finding support and freedom in standing and turning over that leg. After questioning JP about past injuries, he casually mentioned that years ago he had undergone knee surgery on his right knee to repair a torn meniscus, and a few years later had suffered a torn labrum in his right hip joint. He assured me that these past injuries had healed completely and that his strength coach had him squatting and deadlifting large amounts of weight to ensure the strength in the leg. Indeed, he was very strong in his legs in a weight-lifting sense, but he had trouble organizing his movement to stand over the high point of his hip joint and therefore balance effectively in order to perform the skills he needed to employ. This dysfunctional pattern of use was the weak link in his armor.

I worked with JP lying prone over my Feldenkrais table with his knees and lower legs on the floor. In this position, I was able to touch, move, and organize the most proximal parts: his pelvis, ribs, and thoracic spine. What directions of movement of the pelvis in relation to the hip joints did JP need to be able to sense the stability of his anatomic structure and give him the feeling of being able to move in any direction over each leg?

Sitting behind JP, I was able to move his pelvis in all six cardinal directions: forward and backward tilting, side to side, up and down, and rotation left and right. Because the hip joints are not extended in this position, the proprioceptive information is not sensed as in standing, so there is no feeling of threat to previously injured areas. Also, the extensor musculature of his back, serving as the antigravity muscles while upright, were not engaged in this position, which enhanced the kinesthetic communication between the pelvis and the thoracic spine. Eventually JP's ribs softened and his breathing deepened; I then worked with his head, neck, and shoulders, and he became able to laterally flex his spine in both directions. More degrees of freedom had been restored or relearned in his neuromuscular system, and as he returned to standing up he could immediately feel the difference in his improved stability over each leg, and was able to maintain his head free to orient in all directions.

Over the next few days, I worked with JP in a variety of positions, while revisiting this same theme of finding ways to enhance the proprioceptive connection between his pelvis, thorax, and head. At the end of his final session, he was able to move from a quadripedal position to being suspended up and over his right leg/hip and right hand/arm, with his head free to scan the environment. After he returned to the ice, JP reported back to me his newfound ability not only to make tighter turns in his skating patterns but to quickly pause and shoot the puck off either leg. Delighted with this discovery, he immediately set out to find ways to integrate them into his play.

Ecological adaptability and dynamic equilibrium

Human Posture, in spite of the implications of the static "posting," is a dynamic equilibrium. A posture is good if it can regain equilibrium after a large disturbance.

Feldenkrais 1981, p. 43

The focus of my *Functional Integration* movement lessons is this: how can my clients organize the actions necessary for their sport, and can they learn more control and agility in what's commonly called "the core" of the body?

Many improvements in ability have no connection to simply improving strength. For example, if a small child is trying to learn to ride a bike, strapping large weights onto their legs is not going to help them learn new motor control and balance patterns. Unfortunately, although many sports training programs improve muscular strength in certain planes of action, they also increase the internal resistance to movement, thus reducing sensory acuity to anything but the feeling of resistance. This makes it harder to recognize either habits of tension and stress or the unnecessary or parasitic effort with which these are often associated. These habits of resistance reside deep in the tonic musculature, as well as in the musculature around all of our joints. Because of the huge demands they put on themselves in training and performance, professional athletes will be more prone to injury if their deep intrinsic musculature is not well organized for efficient action.

Thus, much of my work consists of observation and exploration, both visually and tactilely, to find the path of least resistance through the skeleton so the client can sense and feel efficiency and grace in his movements – a new sense of spontaneity and agility.

Also, superior equilibrium capacity is required in many sports to attain the greatest competitive level.

The brain and central nervous system integrate visual, vestibular, and proprioceptive data to create motor commands that coordinate muscle patterns of activation in order to regulate equilibrium.

Case Study: CJ – learning to fly again

CJ had previously won an Olympic gold medal in a freestyle skiing event. Now, three years later, she was struggling in the World Cup to regain her prominence and achieve the scores necessary to even qualify for her own national qualifying trials in anticipation of

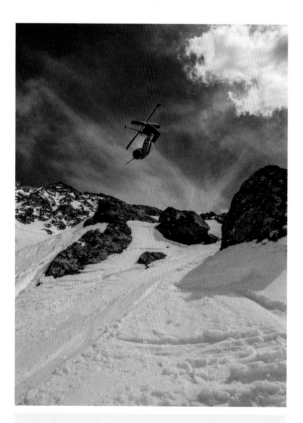

Figure 17.3

Dave Susko @fotophreak

the upcoming Olympic games. When I met CJ, she talked about her lack of confidence and enthusiasm for the sport she had once loved and competed in since she was a young girl. She admitted to a couple of bad falls that had caused probable concussions, but she had kept them secret from the medical staff so she wouldn't be disqualified from the competition.

Now, several years later, it was obvious how spatially compromised she had become. I asked her to jump and turn left and right, first 90 degrees, then 180, and finally a 360-degree jump turn. As expected for an Olympic-level athlete, she performed the jumps enthusiastically and flawlessly, but her landings when she jumped to the left were never quite clear and always a bit wobbly. This tendency was indicative of her current problems in competition, in which she needed to be able to take off in any direction from both or either leg and then launch herself into the air to flip, rotate, spin, and finally land on her skis at high speed, and with elegance.

CJ had a compromised spatial awareness; she was unable to perceive herself in space in certain positions and orientations, like a perceptual "blind spot." Impact injuries, especially multiple impacts that shake the brain, can result in forgetfulness, loss of cognitive ability, vision problems, coordination, and balance deficits. As we worked together, her brain was gradually able to reform the spatial relationships that had become disorganized.

A primary human function is the ability to turn right and left around a vertical axis and to be able to quickly orient to the space around us. In CJ's sport, she was required to do this flawlessly and precisely, but also in a variety of positions and orientations that include doing aerial spins, flips, and even skiing backwards.

In one of our sessions together, CJ lay supine on my Feldenkrais table; I supported her legs with a firm foam roller so that her antigravity extensor muscles would not be engaged in holding her upright. This position serves to reduce the amount of nervous system stimulation, especially from the soles of the feet. Since there are no compressive forces acting on the body in this position, there is a quieting of the normal proprioceptive sensations in the joints and muscles of the ankles, knees, and hips that occur in upright positions. The vestibular system is also quieted down, and the input to the visual cortex is reduced as a client closes their eyes. With this quieting of the habitual input related to normal uprightness, the motor cortex is also freer to sense and form new patterns with minimal input. It is a very comfortable way to lie, as if floating in a saline solution.

I started with touching CJ's right foot with the back of my hand, a relatively flat surface, to determine how she tracked the movement of her foot against the surface of my hand. We had already determined that she was a bit more stable on this leg in standing, so I was supplying some very clear and precise proprioceptive input into her nervous system. After a while, I used my hands to begin to differentiate the skeletal structure of her foot and ankle in relation to standing, slowing the timing of my tactile explorations to coincide with her breathing, which slowed and deepened.

After some time, the movements of her foot and ankle became smoother and I could begin to straighten her leg by pushing with a small amount of compressive force up into her hip via her cuboid. This point of sustentation in relation to our center of gravity is immediately recognized by all humans as being beneficial and a place of clear stability, and the whole system begins to self-organize around this clearer proprioceptive sense.

I moved to sit above her head and began to slowly and softly roll her head left and right, so she could feel the difference in her availability to roll her head to the right, as the neck muscles had become

less tonified and her turning radius had increased dramatically.

After a while, I repeated a similar sequence beginning with her left foot and ankle, sensing that she needed some more time to make the sensory connections on this side. Eventually, I returned to rolling her head; now it traveled much more easily to her left, and the resistance I had felt in her tonic musculature at the beginning had dissipated.

Slowly, I brought her up to sitting so that she could reorient to the space around herself, and then to standing up so that she could feel the change in contact with her feet against the ground. CJ immediately noticed the clearer contact through both feet and her greatly improved ability to turn left and right easily, with much less muscular effort.

I then asked CJ to stand with her hands against the wall with a firm styrofoam roller underneath her left foot. I asked her to slowly roll the roller forward and back, heel to toe, so the movements became smooth and easy instead of the initial jumpiness that occurred. Next, with her left foot still on the roller, I asked CJ to lift her right heel so that she was balanced on the fourth metatarsal of her forefoot. In this position, up over the high point of the hip joint, I asked her to slowly begin turning her head left and right, first with both eyes open, then with one eye closed. After a few repetitions, I asked her to step off the roller and again checked her turning ability left and right, which had improved even more, especially as she turned to the right and shifted her weight over the right leg while turning her head. I asked her to repeat the whole sequence standing with her left foot on the ground, the roller under her right foot, and then eventually with both feet standing on the roller and her hands not touching the wall for support.

In a way, this progression had allowed CJ to feel, sense, and learn a new motor skill that would greatly enhance her ability to function in her world of elite sport competition. She wrote to me months later, after she had qualified again for the upcoming Olympic Games, stating that the awareness she had developed through our sessions together had led her to new ways of practicing and developing new strategies for her training and competition – and she was happy to be able to perform at that level again.

I've presented here some examples of how I utilize the Feldenkrais Method as a comprehensive approach to improving human movement and action outside traditional biomechanical interventions; one that works with the ability for continual adjustment to the environment. In my experience, the method bridges the gap between the science of coaching, rehabilitation, strength conditioning, and recovery, where dexterity, adaptability, and mastery really live.

References

Feldenkrais, M. 1981. *The Elusive Obvious.* Meta Publications, CA.

Feldenkrais, M. 1985. *The Potent Self: A study of spontaneity and compulsion.* Frog Books/Somatic Resources, Berkeley, CA.

Other resources

Bernstein, N. 1967. *The Coordination and Regulation of Movements.* Pergamon Press, Oxford.

Bernstein, N.A. 1996. *Dexterity and Its Development.* L. Erlbaum Associates, Mahwah, NJ.

Latash, M.L. 2012. The bliss (not the problem) of motor abundance (not redundancy). *Experimental Brain Research* 217(1):1–5.

Sherrington, C. 1906. *The Integrative Action of the Nervous System.* Cambridge University Press, Cambridge, UK.

Stuart, D. 2005. Integration of posture and movement: Contributions of Sherrington, Hess, and Bernstein. *Human Movement Science* 24:621–643. doi: 10.1016/j.humov.2005.09.011

The Eyes Organize the Movement of the Body *Awareness Through Movement* Audio Lesson taught by Dwight Pargee

In the last few decades, yoga has experienced explosive growth across the United States and the Western world. According to the 2016 Yoga in America Study (Yoga Alliance 2016), 30 million people in the US practice yoga, mostly asana based. Yoga, however, is much more than asana; it also includes awareness, breath practices, meditation, and more.

The two methods both use movement to learn through the nervous system

In Chapter 1, verse 2 of Patanjali's Yoga Sutras, the line "Chitta Vritti Nirodha" (Aranya 1983), most commonly translated as stilling the waves of the mind, is stated as the goal of yoga. Moshe Feldenkrais often said when training people that he wasn't after flexible bodies, but flexible brains. He was looking for a way to give options about how to act in different contexts and environments, so that we are not ruled by our habits.

One could argue that Feldenkrais' idea about people having options to act differently in different contexts could lead to yoga's quieting of the mind, since a person who has more options has the confidence that they will be able to act appropriately and optimally in any context or environment. One could also argue that once the waves of the mind have slowed down, as in yoga, the person will not feel stressed in unfamiliar environments or contexts, and will therefore act in an appropriate and optimal way. This chapter is not about which approach is better; instead, it aims to suggest how utilizing the Feldenkrais Method can enhance yoga's approach to learning.

The yoga teacher needs to keep in mind that the two approaches differ, so it is not simply about making random movement variations. The idea is to set up intentional differentiation and constraints that are congruent with earlier movements and that will challenge the nervous system to find new (movement) solutions. Before we look at differentiation and constraints, let's look at how yoga asanas can introduce learning through the nervous system and what the limitations of regular asana practice may be.

While both yoga and the Feldenkrais Method include movement and awareness that can modulate and change the nervous system, yoga's popularity has taken off in a way that the Feldenkrais Method has not. Before we delve into how the principles of Feldenkrais can enhance yoga practice, let's look at the history of yoga and how it managed to grow at such an astonishing rate compared to the Feldenkrais Method.

History of yoga in the United States

Yoga was introduced to the United States in 1893, when Swami Vivekananda made a presentation of yoga as a spiritual practice in Chicago at the World Parliament of Religions (Shaw 2010). It continued to be considered mostly a spiritual practice in the US until Richard Hittleman emphasized the physical benefits in the 1950s (Kent 1972), at about the same time as Jack LaLanne started his eponymous television show (which ran until 1985) to capture the growing interest in physical practice in the United States.

In the 1960s and 70s, yoga connected to many popular cultural events: Swami Satchidananda opened the Woodstock Festival in 1969; Ram Dass toured college campuses; and Transcendental Meditation spread throughout the United States. Influential teachers such as B.K.S. Iyengar, Pattabhi Joyce, and T.K.V. Desikachar taught in the US. Many of these events introduced and connected yoga and popular music to what was known as the hippie generation.

Since that time, yoga has continued to attract influential figures in music, acting and athletics. Examples of people who practice yoga include Madonna, Sting, Robert Downey Jr., Lady Gaga, David Beckham, and LeBron James, as well as professional teams like the Seattle Seahawks. This has kept yoga in the media spotlight and allowed it to continue to grow and develop a certain kind of "coolness."

As yoga has grown, so has the business of yoga grown. In 2017 the US yoga business was valued at $16.8 billion (Yoga Alliance 2020). It is not uncommon, these days, for airports and hotels to have yoga rooms where travelers can practice. The US-based Yoga Alliance, formed in 1999 as an organization for yoga teachers and yoga schools, has over 100,000 individual members and over 6,000 school members (Yoga Alliance 2020). So, while the title of this chapter is "Feldenkrais to Enhance Yoga," we should also examine how yoga can enhance and help the Feldenkrais Method grow. Both yoga and Feldenkrais use movement as a way to learn through the nervous system, but they do it in different ways.

Yoga as a modality for learning through the nervous system

Many common asanas, such as Downward Dog (Figure 18.1), put the student in a body alignment where their proprioceptors are out of alignment. In such a situation, the student's nervous system has to *figure out how to maintain balance and stability*. In addition, in Downward Dog, the student has to bear weight on the hands, something that most people are not used to doing. This forces the student's nervous system to figure out how to maintain stability in the pose and eventually transition out of that pose and into the next one. It challenges

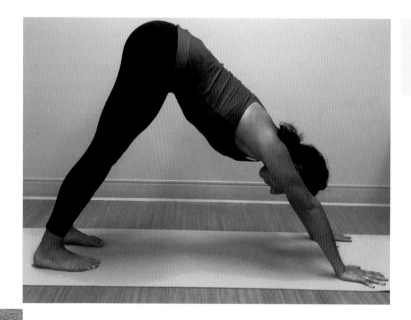

Figure 18.1
Downward Dog pose.

Courtesy of Staffan Elgelid

the student, but with repeated practice, the poses become familiar. The student gets into the habit of how to perform the asanas, how one asana follows the next, and the pace of the sequence. After a while, however, the nervous system loses interest and minimal learning takes place.

How can the Feldenkrais Method enhance the asana practice so that learning through the nervous system continues?

How to use the principles of the Feldenkrais Method in yoga

The Feldenkrais Method is a type of somatic education and, as such, the body is considered the primary vehicle for learning. Observe when an infant learns a new skill, such as crawling or walking; the child will try each skill in a multitude of different ways. Once sufficient proficiency has been acquired to reach the goal for the action, the infant will perform it repeatedly, but with fewer variations. It is not until they need to improve the skill to reach a new goal, or learn a new skill, that large variations in the movement occur again. As we get older, we tend to perform a familiar skill the same way repeatedly, because it has become habitual and learning has more or less ceased. It does not, however, mean that we cannot learn new skills.

Differentiation and constraints

In the Feldenkrais Method, differentiation and constraints are deliberately incorporated into the movement explorations. The Feldenkrais practitioner uses them to set up a movement that challenges the student's nervous system to find new ways of performing a specific skill or action. The differentiation and constraints vary, depending on the habitual movement patterns of the student that would benefit from being revised.

Creating differentiation

The Feldenkrais concept of differentiation can be applied to yoga asanas in several ways, during the asana or during the transition between asanas. The differentiation can be in where the movement is initiated, how the breathing is incorporated into it, the flow of its different aspects, or how it is paced, as well as in other aspects of the asana practice.

Today many yoga teachers are beginning to break down asanas (commonly in ways that are based on biomechanical principles), with the intention of creating variations that prevent injuries. The way the Feldenkrais Method differentiates, however, is based more on the nervous system and learning. The differentiation must occur in a way that makes sense to the nervous system, so that the student can connect it to the previous movement. Here are some brief examples of how to differentiate the transition from Mountain pose to Warrior I pose and back to Mountain. These examples could easily be used in the transition between any asanas and can be incorporated into any yoga asana sequence.

Differentiation of the initiation of movement

Finding the habitual movement:

1 Start by standing in Mountain pose with the feet hip-width apart and the arms relaxed alongside your body (Figure 18.2).

2 Transition from Mountain pose to Warrior I, stepping back with the left leg (Figure 18.3).

3 Transition back to Mountain pose from Warrior I.

4 Reflect on where you initiated the movement as you transitioned from Mountain to Warrior I and then back to Mountain. Were you aware of what part of you initiated each movement?

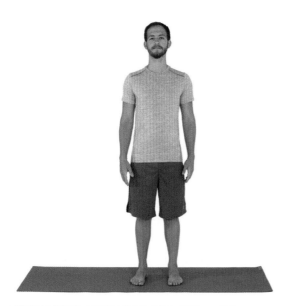

Figure 18.2
Mountain pose.

Courtesy of and © Human Kinetics

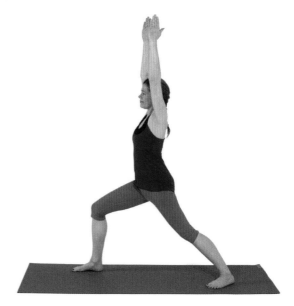

Figure 18.3
Warrior I pose.

Courtesy of and © Human Kinetics

5 Do the same sequence, now paying attention to where you initiated the movement. This is your habitual way of transitioning from Mountain to Warrior I and back to Mountain.

Now that you have identified your habitual way of transitioning between those asanas, try to differentiate the initiation of the movement.

Differentiation 1

1 Start by standing in Mountain pose with the feet hip-width apart and the arms relaxed alongside your body.

2 Transition from Mountain pose to Warrior I by initiating the movement from the left arm, and then let the rest of the body follow.

3 Transition back to Mountain pose from Warrior I, still initiating the movement from the left arm.

Differentiation 2

As above, but now initiate the movement from the *pelvis* as you transition between the poses.

Differentiation 3

As above, but now initiate the movement from the *head* as you transition between the poses.

Differentiation 4

As above, but now initiate the movement from the *left foot* as you transition between the poses.

Differentiation 5

As above, but now initiate the movement from the *left foot*, then turn the *pelvis*, then the *left arm*, and finally the *head* when you transition from Mountain pose to Warrior I. Follow the same initiation and sequence of the movement as you transition back to Mountain pose. This transition is focusing on the initiation of the movement as well as the sequence through the body.

Differentiation 6

As above, but now initiate the movement from the *head*, then the *left arm*, then the *pelvis*, and finally the *left foot* when you transition from Mountain pose to Warrior I. Follow the same initiation and sequence of the movement as you transition back to Mountain pose.

Integration

1 Stand in Mountain pose. Do you feel a difference between the left and right side of the body? Do you feel a difference in how you contact the ground between the two feet?

2 Do the original transition from Mountain pose to Warrior I back to Mountain pose. Did the movement change? Did the place you initiated the movement from change? Are you more aware of where the movement initiates, the sequence of the movement through the body, and how you transition between the asanas?

Differentiation of the breath and the coordination between the breath and the movement

Finding the habitual breath pattern:

1 Start by standing in Mountain pose with the feet hip-width apart and the arms relaxed alongside your body.

2 Transition from Mountain pose to Warrior I, stepping back with the left leg.

3 Transition back to Mountain pose from Warrior I.

4 Reflect on whether you were *breathing in* or *out* or *holding the breath* as you transitioned between the poses. Were you aware of your breathing as you moved?

5 Do the same sequence, now paying attention to your breathing. This is your habitual way to breathe as you transition between the poses.

Differentiation 1

As above, but *breathe in* as you transition from Mountain pose to Warrior I; stay in Warrior I for one breath cycle and then transition back to Mountain on your *out-breath*.

Differentiation 2

As above, but *breathe out* as you transition from Mountain pose to Warrior I; stay in Warrior I for one breath cycle, and then transition back to Mountain on your *in-breath*.

Differentiation 3

As above, but *hold your breath* as you transition from Mountain pose to Warrior I; stay in Warrior I for one breath cycle and then transition back to Mountain *holding your breath*.

Integration

1 Stand in Mountain pose. Are you more aware of your breath? Do you feel a difference in how you contact the ground?

2 Do the original transition between the poses. Did the movement or breathing change? Are you more aware of how you breathe during the transitions?

Differentiating by setting up incongruencies

Differentiation 1

As above, but *slow down* your breathing, so that you are breathing half as fast as normal. Allow the breath to stabilize at the slower rate, then move quickly from Mountain to Warrior I and back to Mountain. Do several of these transition cycles rapidly while you are maintaining the slow breath.

Differentiation 2

As above, but *increase the rate of breathing*, so that you are breathing twice as fast as normal. Allow the breath to stabilize at the faster rate, then move very slowly from Mountain to Warrior I and back to Mountain. Do several of these transition cycles slowly while you are maintaining the faster breath.

Integration

1 Stand in Mountain. Are you more aware of your breath? Do you feel a difference in how you contact the ground?

2 Do the original transition between the asanas. Did the movement and breathing change? Are you more aware of how you breathe during the transitions?

The last two variations are very challenging for the nervous system, since it is not "normal" to move fast and breathe slowly, or to move slowly and breathe fast. This sets up an incongruency in the nervous system. Usually when we move fast, we also breathe fast, since it tends to mean we are in a fight or flight situation. When we move slowly and breathe slowly, we are usually in a rest and renew situation. By taking one aspect from fight or flight and another from rest and renew, an incongruency is set up in the nervous system and the nervous system has to solve the puzzle.

Setting up constraints

Another way that ideas from the Feldenkrais Method can enhance yoga is through setting up constraints. Differentiation is a kind of constraint, but there are more obvious ways to set up constraints in asana practice.

Cat and Cow is a common asana that is usually practiced early on as a warm-up pose.

Finding the habitual movement:

1 The student begins on hands and knees.

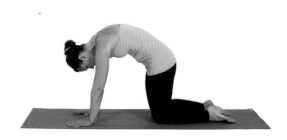

Figure 18.4
Cat pose.

Courtesy of and © Human Kinetics

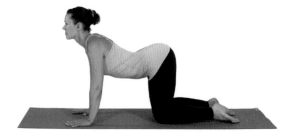

Figure 18.5
Cow pose.

Courtesy of and © Human Kinetics

2 The student goes back and forth between rounding the back up toward the ceiling (cat; Figure 18.4) and letting the spine drop toward the floor (cow; Figure 18.5).

3 After the student has performed the movement in the habitual way and noticed how they are doing the movement, the teacher can set up constraints based on their observation of how the student performed the asana.

Constraint 1

As the student performs the asana, ask them to hold the lumbar spine in neutral. All the movements will then occur in the thoracic and cervical spine.

Constraint 2

Ask the student to hold the cervical spine in neutral, so that all the movement occurs in the thoracic and lumbar spine.

Constraint 3

Ask the student to assume Child's pose and transition into Cat and Cow from that position. This will limit the amount of movement that can occur in the lumbar spine, so more movement will take place in the thoracic spine.

Constraints can be set up in a variety of ways and in any asana or transition between asanas.

How can the Feldenkrais Method learn from yoga?

Yoga has managed to tap into the fitness trend, something that the Feldenkrais Method has not yet achieved. According to Moti Nativ,[1] Feldenkrais lessons in the 1950s were taken by younger people, who were fit and healthy, which resulted in the lessons being more challenging and difficult. Today's lessons, which are easier (though maybe more effective), do not attract young students who are looking for more strength or flexibility.

Many yoga students feel like they are getting stronger and more flexible when they practice. Improved strength and flexibility is something that is easy for people to understand, and they have the "scaffolding" around the concepts of strength and flexibility. They can talk to friends and neighbors about it. What happens in a Feldenkrais lesson is more subtle. Students feel "different": something happened, but it is difficult to put it into words. They did not strain and did not work on flexibility, but nevertheless, something interesting happened and they feel and move better. Changes in the nervous system are subtle and hard to explain.

If Feldenkrais practitioners can tie the concepts of strength, flexibility, and fitness together with the concept of learning through the nervous system, there is no reason why the Feldenkrais Method shouldn't become as popular as yoga.

Conclusion

Yoga has experienced incredible growth throughout the Western world, but with that growth there has also been an increase in injuries among people who practice it. By using the Feldenkrais Method's approach of *Awareness Through Movement* as well as the concepts of differentiation and constraints, asana practice can be made safer and allow the nervous system to continue to create new options on how to move and relate in different contexts, leading to an improved ability to thrive in life.

References

Aranya, H. 1983. *Yoga Philosophy of Patanjali*. State University of New York Press, Albany, NY.

1 At the "Feldenkrais and the Martial Arts" workshop held in Amsterdam from February 16 to 19, 2019.

Kent, H. 1972. Yoga for Health: A breakthrough in television programs. In: R. Hutchinson (ed.) *Yoga and Health*. Astrian, London.

Shaw, E. 2010. From the Caves of India to the White House Lawn, Yoga Journal Celebrates 6,000 Years of Practice in 35 Moments. *Yoga Journal* 231:88–96.

Yoga Alliance 2016. Yoga in America Study 2016. *Yoga Journal and Yoga Alliance*. https://www.yogaalliance.org/2016YogaInAmericaStudy [Accessed October, 2020].

Yoga Alliance 2020. https://www.yogaalliance.org [Accessed October, 2020].

Other resources

Bosch, F. 2015. *Strength Training and Coordination: An integrative approach*, translated by Kevin Cook. 2010 Publishers, Rotterdam.

Butera, K., Elgelid, S. 2017. *Yoga Therapy: A personalized approach for your active lifestyle*. Human Kinetics, Champaign, IL.

Claxton, G. 2015. *Intelligence in the flesh: Why your mind needs your body more than it thinks*. Yale University Press, New Haven, CT.

Doidge, N. 2007. *The Brain that Changes Itself: Stories of personal triumph from the frontiers of brain science*. Viking Books, New York.

Doidge, N. 2015. *The Brain's Way of Healing: Remarkable discoveries and recoveries from the frontiers of neuroplasticity*. Viking Books, New York.

Eddy, M. 2016. *Mindful Movement: The evolution of the somatic arts and conscious action*. Intellect, Bristol, UK.

Epstein, D. 2019. *Range: Why generalists triumph in a specialized world*. Riverhead Books, New York.

Hargrove, T.R. 2014. *A Guide to Better Movement: The science and practice of moving with more skill and less pain*. Seattle, WA.

Rywerant, Y. 1983. *The Feldenkrais Method: Teaching by handling*. Keats Publishing, New Canaan, CT.

Awareness Through Movement Audio Lessons taught by Staffan Elgelid

18.1 *Mountain to Warrior 1 with Initiation Differentiations*

18.2 *Mountain to Warrior 1 with Breathing Differentiations*

On first glance, no two movement disciplines seem to have less in common than Feldenkrais and Pilates. With its focus on gentle exploration, a Feldenkrais lesson feels worlds apart from a Pilates exercise session. And while both practices aim to improve health by optimizing movement, the Feldenkrais Method tends to be associated with flexibility, relaxation, and coordination, while Pilates is more often associated with strength, power, and endurance.

The most obvious difference between the two methods is how familiar they are to the general public. With thousands of teachers worldwide and studios throughout the world, Pilates is a brand of exercise most people recognize. Even though Feldenkrais has a roster of over 10,000 certified practitioners worldwide, it is much less visible, and less understood. One reason for this is historical: Pilates predates Feldenkrais by several decades. A second reason is that Moshe Feldenkrais and his followers thoroughly documented and protected his work, whereas Joseph Pilates passed away before this could be done, with the result that the Pilates Method has been widely interpreted and elaborated upon.

This chapter explores each method's approach to learning through the neuromuscular system and demonstrates how they can be used in tandem to optimize well-being. The three case studies show how Feldenkrais can become an adjunct for improving strength, power, and endurance.

Two pioneers

Even though Joseph Pilates and Moshe Feldenkrais developed their methods at different times and in different parts of the world, their paths and journeys of discovery had much in common, in that they both embarked on self-exploration in an effort to overcome debilitating health conditions. Both sought out alternative therapies and familiarized themselves with Eastern mind-body disciplines. Both trained as athletes and engaged in competitive sports. And both took a holistic approach to fitness and well-being.

Joseph Pilates

Pilates was born into a poor Prussian family in 1883. His father was a prize-winning gymnast from Greece and his mother a naturopath of German descent. Like many underprivileged children of the time, he grew up sickly, suffering from rickets, asthma, and rheumatic fever. These ailments took a toll on his size and development, but they also stimulated his early interest in self-improvement and movement. As a child, he was fascinated by the way animals move and accompanied his hard-working father to the local gymnastics club, where he exercised to bolster his health. His father taught him how to box, and he took a liking to it, even though the sport was prohibited in Germany at the time.

By his 20s, Pilates had developed into a competitive boxer and athlete. Along with his self-prescribed fitness routines, he explored martial arts, yoga, and Zen meditation. At the age of 31, he joined a traveling German circus and toured Great Britain, where he could legally box. The outbreak of World War I radically changed his plans, when he and the rest of troupe were forced into a British internment camp on the Isle of Man.

During his four years of confinement, Pilates worked as an orderly in the camp hospital and read extensively about anatomy and physical medicine. He maintained his exercise routines and encouraged other detainees to use his program to preserve their physical and mental health during internment. Pilates even attached springs to hospital beds so patients could benefit from exercise.

When he was repatriated to Germany after the war, Pilates took his progressive ideas of whole-body exercise further. He evolved his exercises to make them more accessible, and prototyped fitness equipment that followed his ideas. Post-war America was a fertile ground for new ideas and in 1926, Pilates immigrated to the US to introduce and expand on his work. He called his exercise system Contrology and established a studio in New York City (Larkam 2017, p. 33). His method quickly caught on among high achievers in the creative arts, with luminaries like Martha Graham and Yehudi Menuhin seeking him out. He published two books, *Your Health: A Corrective System of Exercising That Revolutionizes the Entire Field of Physical Education* and *Return to Life Through Contrology*. He continued teaching throughout his life until his death in 1967 (Pilatesmethodalliance 2013).

Moshe Feldenkrais

Moshe Feldenkrais was born into an orthodox Jewish–Ukrainian family in 1904 – a generation later than Pilates. His father was a rabbi, and throughout his youth, Feldenkrais chafed under the strict Hassidic rules imposed by the community. Highly athletic and self-taught in survival skills, Feldenkrais instructed Palestinian Jews in self-defense. He added jiu-jitsu to his repertoire and was an avid soccer player until he was sidelined with a knee injury. Relentlessly curious about the workings of the mind, Feldenkrais also became interested in hypnosis and Émile Coué's system of autosuggestion.

In the 1930s he relocated to Paris, where he graduated from college with mechanical and electrical engineering degrees. He earned his Doctorate in Physics at the Sorbonne, and continued with post-doctorate studies, working closely with one of his mentors, Nobel Prize laureate Frederic Joliot-Curie (Reese 2015). While in Paris, Feldenkrais' fascination with martial arts led him to study with Professor Jigaro Kano, the founder of judo.

At the outbreak of World War II, Feldenkrais fled Paris to evade the Nazis, and put his education to work on anti-submarine research for Great Britain. He severely reinjured his knee on a submarine deck during this time and was told he would never walk normally again. Undaunted, he turned his engineering skills on the problem. Using himself as the subject, he developed a series of guided movement sequences to help rehabilitate his knee – work that eventually led to the Feldenkrais Method.

By the mid-1950s, he had given up his career in physics to devote himself full-time to the study of human movement. His work began to attract an international following of artists and academics, among them being Yehudi Menuhin, Margaret Mead, and Karl Pribram. His following grew as he conducted seminars and shared his work through multiple writings: *Body and Mature Behavior, Awareness Through Movement, The Case of Nora, The Elusive Obvious, The Master Moves*, and, posthumously, *The Potent Self*. His early students transcribed his teachings to preserve their spirit and intent, and today, many hours of his lessons are still available to students through the International Feldenkrais Federation and the Feldenkrais Guild of North America.

One vision; two paths

The separate paths these two pioneers took a generation apart converge in their belief that overall physical and mental health depend on the ability to move freely throughout life. They developed unique movement education systems based on different kinds of mental and physical engagement.

Pilates: working against resistance – mind over matter

The Pilates Method is a directive and prescriptive system of movement education. Instructors cue students through various equipment or mat-based resistance exercises, encouraging correct form, controlled repetition, and a coordinated breathing technique derived from yoga (Eddy 2009). During a session, Pilates instructors frequently model correct form and guide students with their touch to help isolate and engage the muscle groups targeted in each exercise.

The keys to correct Pilates form are knowing the purpose and mechanism of each exercise, choosing an appropriate level of resistance, and using *psychophysical cues* of centering, concentration, and control. To help students achieve that, Pilates advocated his Contrology system, a kind of *mind-body discipline*. The purpose of Contrology was to focus the mind on the central muscles of the torso, which he called the powerhouse, in order to aggregate heavy workloads.

While these techniques to build strength and endurance were of obvious benefit to the gymnasts, acrobats, and dancers who sought him out, Pilates viewed the underlying principles of his work as being universally applicable.

In order that one may receive the maximum benefit and resulting normal health from one's daily activities, one should understand at least some of the rudimentary underlying principles governing the mechanism of the human body in motion, rest and sleep. For example, knowledge of the leverage possibilities of the skeletal framework, the range and limitation of proper muscle tension and relaxation,

the laws of equilibrium and gravity, and last but not least, how to inhale and exhale (i.e., how to breathe properly and normally), are essential if we are to benefit from any exercises.

Larkam 2017, p. 31

While the term Contrology has largely faded from use, Pilates's belief in the importance of mindful engagement during exercise has been widely adopted by today's somatically oriented Pilates instructors.

Feldenkrais: working toward efficiency

Feldenkrais took a different approach to resistance and the role of awareness in his system of movement education. Instead of focusing on external resistance to load and unload muscle groups as Pilates did, Feldenkrais focused on patterns of resistance within our own bodies that inhibit fluid movement or cause pain. He believed that many of these debilitating patterns are deeply ingrained in us and are either difficult to detect or unconscious. Feldenkrais used awareness through gentle touch or verbal suggestion to heighten kinesthetic sensitivity, reveal these patterns of resistance, and facilitate a more even distribution of effort throughout the body.

Feldenkrais developed two learning strategies to achieve those objectives: *Functional Integration* (FI) and *Awareness Through Movement* (ATM). In an FI session, practitioners use gentle touch to discover areas of internal resistance and explore alternate pathways to attenuate pain and improve overall organization. In ATM lessons, teachers verbally guide students through a series of gentle, exploratory exercises that progressively build awareness and improve movement efficiency. Teachers encourage students to do these structured sequences slowly and deliberately, so the body can sense small variations. Feldenkrais did not advocate any specific form of breathing, but his lessons are designed to uncover, and provide alternatives to, habits that interfere with the flow of breath.

Although Feldenkrais frequently referred to the process of organizing and refining movement through FI or ATM as creating a more accurate "body map" (or image) based on new information, each student's map is different. Each person's learning is based on their own experience of what works and what doesn't. The Feldenkrais Method is neither corrective nor prescriptive in this regard. In fact, Feldenkrais encouraged his students to learn as children do – not by imitating forms of movement, but by experimenting and eventually discovering how the human body is wired to crawl and walk, sit and stand, along with all the other wonderful things it is capable of.

While Feldenkrais did not develop dedicated equipment as part of his somatic practice, he was well known for using the floor, chairs, and everyday tools to help clients become aware of their movement patterns. One repurposed tool he came to rely on was the foam roller (Figure 19.1). He began

exploring rollers after he saw solid wooden cylinders being used to move heavy equipment. Feldenkrais used firm cardboard and foam rollers to create new conditions for learning in an ever-changing environment. Rollers offered him dynamic ways to tune the body to be more receptive – they were his way of facilitating childlike learning through curiosity, exploration, and play.

Exercising choices – Feldenkrais as foundation

Feldenkrais often said, *"If you know what you are doing, you can do what you want"* (Feldenkrais 1995), and the concept behind that simple phrase is one of the tenets of his work. Having a refined awareness of what you are doing frees you from being driven by compulsive or unconscious habits.

As a physical therapist, I spent years learning through continuing education and patient care, but the Feldenkrais Method offered me my first opportunity to learn through direct experience. What I learned in the training through my own movement was that the Feldenkrais approach to sensorimotor learning is a powerful springboard to more mature and refined movements of all kinds – from playing the violin to running a marathon. When the body is attuned to recognize optimum balance in different positions, posture becomes dynamic and more adaptable to the action at hand, whether that is getting up from a chair to walk across a room or moving rocks to build a wall.

The Feldenkrais Method also catalyzed my interest in other models of somatic education, particularly Pilates. The Pilates Method is often recommended as a rehabilitation program – most commonly for back problems – but most Pilates instructors would agree that before embarking on any kind of therapeutic exercise, clients must learn how to move *without* pain or risk of re-injury. Feldenkrais can be a foundation for that.

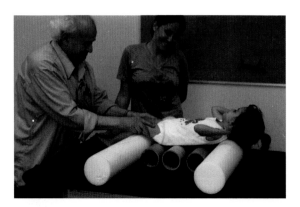

Figure 19.1
Moshe Feldenkrais using rollers to work with a child.

Case Study 1: amateur triathlete

I was approached by a skilled triathlete whose recent fall had left him with severe low back pain radiating down his left leg. To avoid surgery, his surgeon had referred him to a clinic that put him on a rigorous rehabilitation program of stretching and progressive lumbar stabilization exercises combined with manual therapy. Despite having followed this program diligently for a few months, he saw little improvement and was unable to return to sports.

On his first visit, I noticed that, despite being athletic, his movement visibly aged him. He walked with a rigid pelvis, had little trunk rotation, and his chest was so restricted that it compromised his ability to breathe. Although he had more strength than most people, he had limited functional mobility and spoke of feeling old and disabled. He was only 30 years old.

He had a great reserve of athletic ability, but he couldn't find it. From what I could see, his map of his own body seemed to be inaccurate, as if his GPS coordinates were off.

We started our work together with an FI lesson that encouraged him to let go of areas in his body he was unconsciously clenching. That jump-started his kinesthetic re-mapping, and from there we added ATMs to help him refine his neuromuscular awareness. Next, we added a foam roller to his routine. This heightened his ability to discriminate by progressively training his kinesthetic sense in ever-changing positions. (Refer to the *Roller* lesson audio file at the end of this chapter.)

Before the client could return to strength and endurance training, we needed to make sure he was organized for more dynamic movement. We used a Feldenkrais imagery strategy called the "Five Lines"

to create a three-dimensional reference he could easily access when he returned to more demanding activities.

By this time, he was ready for Pilates exercises. These less exploratory, more prescriptive exercises complemented the Feldenkrais Method by engaging the right amount of resistance for his ability.

It was time to test his movement awareness with even higher loads: starting with light workouts in the pool before progressing to running short distances at first, and then adding miles and speed as he absorbed the new body-mapping information. As his workouts ramped up, he continued doing ATMs to improve his dynamic alignment and coordination. He also sought advice from Feldenkrais practitioner Edward Yu to improve his running form. Soon, we were comfortable referring him to a Pilates studio that aligned with our somatic philosophy and plan of care.

Four months later, this once-compromised athlete was able to compete in and finish one of America's most grueling endurance events: the Alcatraz Triathlon.

Every client has different goals, needs, and capacities. This client's recovery story would not be possible had he not had an open mind and been intensely dedicated to his own rehabilitation. For all these reasons, his case study shouldn't be taken as a formula for success, but as one illustration of how Feldenkrais and Pilates can be used together to reach a specific goal.

Case Study 2: active senior

The general strategy of helping clients refine their movement awareness to reach a specific goal does not just apply to athletes. It can be used with clients whose starting points and goals are much more modest.

An elderly client I worked with suffered from visual deficits and a paralyzing fear of falling. She had also been diagnosed with bone-density loss and was concerned about the risk of fractures as she aged. Her fears had compromised her functional mobility so severely that she lacked the confidence to continue attending her seniors exercise classes.

We began our work together with an FI lesson designed to get her to feel more stable and at less risk of falling. After her first session, we gave her a Feldenkrais-inspired home program that included short, recorded ATMs for overall movement awareness, plus a Wall-Spinal Chain exercise that explores slow spinal segment-by-segment movement (Figure 19.2). The goal was to help her experience how coordinated spinal movements affected her sense of balance and support. By reducing her fear and improving her trunk flexibility, she could react more spontaneously to balance challenges. (Refer to the *Spine as a Chain* audio file at the end of this chapter.)

The second FI built on the client's improved awareness and allowed us to introduce gentle Pilates leg circle exercises on the Cadillac (Figure 19.3). I elevated her torso and head with a foam wedge to provide safe support and used light springs to help her access hip and pelvic control.

When she stood up after the leg circles, she was more aware of her hips and pelvic floor and felt a clearer understanding of their role in her structural support and balance. Prior to the exercise, she had felt a weakness in her pelvic floor area and was amazed that she could feel improvement in this without setting it as a goal.

After a short period, she was able to return to her Qi Gong and Pilates classes. Despite her visual

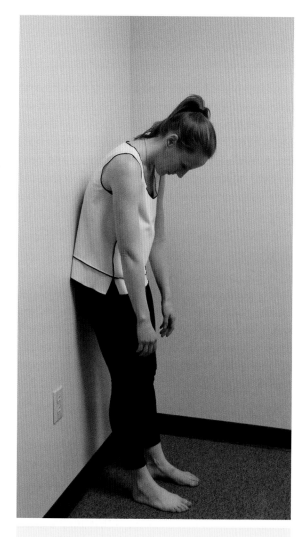

Figure 19.2
Wall-Spinal Chain exercise.

Courtesy of Stacy Barrows

deficits, she now had the internal sense of balance that allowed her to participate without fear of falling. She resumed an active, independent lifestyle that included gravity-based exercises to help her avoid further bone loss. With her new-found ability to be more active, the client also became

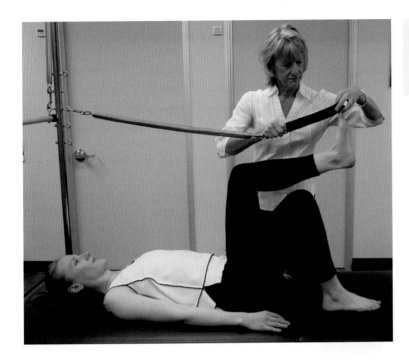

Figure 19.3
Cadillac exercise.

Courtesy of Stacy Barrows

happier with her appearance and more confident in her movement generally.

Case Study 3: aspiring dancer

Somatic practitioners routinely see clients suffering from a condition known medically as multisystem connective tissue disorder or hypermobility syndrome (Sahin, Atik, and Sargin 2015, p. 1). People with this condition have excessive play in their joints, particularly their shoulders and hips. When they load these unstable joints through their arms and legs, it can cause joint discomfort or neck and back pain. Frequent stretching to temporarily relieve the discomfort may only compound the problem, and even diligent core training often has little effect on the underlying structural problem.

A dancer in her mid-20s came to me with debilitating pain related to hypermobility. She had tried frequent stretching and several types of exercise to no avail, and her frustration had led her to give up dancing entirely.

On her first visit, I immediately noticed her lack of fine motor control. In addition, her joints seemed extremely loose and unstable; her arms and legs did not seem integrated with the rest of her body. Even simple movements with almost no load on her extremities took her to the end range of her joints. She was by all measures flexible and strong, but her joints were overworked. She was habitually engaging her musculoskeletal system in ways that contributed to her pain and discomfort.

We began to help her refine her movement awareness so she could move in a more coordinated, comfortable manner. Several FIs helped her find alternative ways to move her limbs – using better skeletal support to help relieve the stress on her joints. The FIs also expanded her sensation of movement to areas of her body that she was

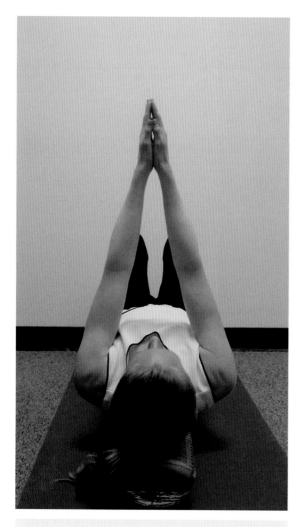

Figure 19.4
Awareness Through Movement on a Smartroller.

Courtesy of Stacy Barrows

at finding neutral joint positions when she placed light loads on her extremities. (Refer to the *Five Lines* audio file at the end of this chapter.)

With better joint centration and more awareness of her own movement, she was ready to test variable load conditions on the Pilates equipment.

This progression of exercise brought about a dramatic change in her comfort and mood. While her pain did not completely disappear, its frequency and intensity lessened sufficiently for her to return to dancing. She also returned to her Pilates classes to continue building strength and endurance, and added mini-Feldenkrais lessons to prepare for her classes. Her somatic explorations gave her a renewed sense of her body in space and a more confident self-image; and she now has the tools she needs to manage her own symptoms.

Conclusion

Using the Feldenkrais Method as a foundation for refined movement has broad application. While this chapter demonstrated its use along with Pilates to help a triathlete, senior, and dancer reach their unique goals, the Feldenkrais process of building awareness, seeking even distribution of effort and developing a more accurate body map can benefit anyone who wants to move well in their daily activities. Whether those activities are as simple as standing or sitting, or as complex as weightlifting, playing a fugue, or throwing an opponent in judo, Feldenkrais helps people develop a level of competency and refinement that can enhance any performance.

While Feldenkrais and Pilates each address the issues of resistance and mental engagement in their own unique ways, both leverage the human body's limitless potential for learning and growth to achieve lasting outcomes.

previously unaware of, particularly her jaw and spine. We carried this whole-body awareness-building strategy forward with a home program of ATMs. This included the "Five Lines" lesson to help her systematically visualize where she was directing force in her body when she initiated movement. As she refined her body map, she became more skilled

References

(*My gratitude to Pilates and somatic experts Sonia Kissel, Rael Isacowitz, Trina Altman, Amy Alpers, Risa Sheppard, Brenda Provo, Kelly Haney, Dr Martha Eddy, and Elizabeth Larkam.*)

Eddy, M. 2009. A Brief History of Somatic Practices and Dance: Historical development of the field of somatic education and its relationship to dance. *Journal of Dance and Somatic Practices* 1(1):5–27. Available at: www.wellnesscke.net

Feldenkrais, M. 1995. *Dr. Moshe Feldenkrais at Alexander Yanai,* Vols. 1–12. International Feldenkrais Federation, Paris.

Larkam, E. 2017. *Fascia in Motion.* Kindle edition. Handspring, UK.

Pilatesmethodalliance 2013. "The History of Pilates" https://pilatesmethodalliance.org/PMA/About/History-of-Pilates/PMA/About/History-of-Pilates.aspx?hkey=fd57cd07-4353-481d-818e-25a0007d5de6 [Accessed October 27, 2020].

Reese, M. 2015. *Moshe Feldenkrais: A life in movement.* ReeseKress Somatics Press, San Rafael, CA.

Sahin, N., Atik, A., Sargin, S. 2015. Joint hypermobility syndrome and related pain. *Archives of Clinical Experimental Surgery* 5(3):1. doi:10.5455/aces.20150508124321 https://www.researchgate.net/publication/276458194

Other resources

Yu, E. 2012. *Slowing Down Faster,* http://slowingdownfaster.com

Awareness Through Movement Audio Lessons taught by Stacy Barrows		
19.1	*Roller*	
19.2	*Spine as a Chain*	
19.3	*Five Lines*	

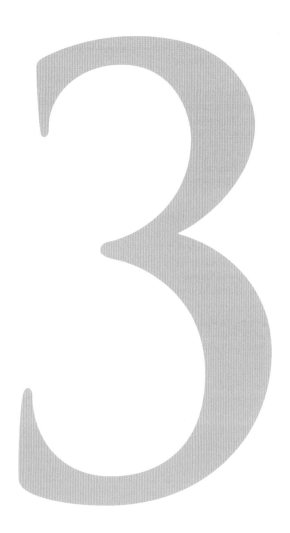

During the first year of the Amherst training, Moshe Feldenkrais said that he worked with people's health rather than their illness or diagnosis. Based on this comment, it may seem strange to include a chapter on how to use the Feldenkrais Method to deal with orthopedic problems, but as we will see, the principles of the Feldenkrais Method can truly enhance the way rehab professionals work with orthopedic clients.

The word orthopedics comes from the Greek root word ortho – meaning straight. Traditionally, orthopedic rehabilitation interventions have involved rehab techniques including stretching, strengthening, and a variety of modalities such as ice and heat. These approaches have worked reasonably well, but many patients never quite recover from their injuries, or at least not to pre-injury functioning. The patients continue to complain about nagging aches and pains and sustain repeated injuries.

Having worked as a physical therapist for more than 30 years, it is clear to me that we need a new approach to the rehabilitation of orthopedic injuries so that the client can return to full pre-injury status and avoid their recurrence. Persistent pain is discussed in Chapter 22, so this chapter will focus on how the Feldenkrais Method can complement and improve orthopedic rehabilitation.

In today's rehab climate, clients are being seen for fewer sessions and shorter periods of time per session. I have therefore simplified my process in the case study to make it more practical for rehab professionals who are limited in the amount of time they have available to see their patients.

Case Study

The female client was a former college athlete in her late 20s who had a series of right ankle sprains while still in college. Since then, she had remained actively involved in sports but continued to suffer from ankle sprains, stress fractures in the right foot, and overuse injuries in the left leg. The client had undergone several sessions of physical therapy, consisting of stretching, strengthening, and balance exercises, before she contacted me.

It was clear that more stretching, strengthening, and balance rehab would not help this client, since there were no deficits in those areas. What I did notice was that she put more weight on the left leg, and that her whole body was shifted toward the left side. From a Feldenkrais perspective this made sense. When we get injured, the nervous system is trying to protect us from pain. The nervous system is trying to find a pain-free way to accomplish all the movements and functions that the person normally performs, and often the whole body shifts away from the painful area. But sometimes the nervous system does too good a job protecting us from pain and does not stop protecting us once the injury has healed.

In the case of this client, it meant putting more weight on the left foot/leg, and, by the time I saw her, the nervous system had adopted that as the "new normal." The muscles in the left leg and that side of the body, therefore, had to work harder.

Session 1. Noticing the weight shift
During the first session, the majority of the time was spent working on having the client noticing

how she put more weight on the left leg and how that impacted the whole left side of her body. For a client to be able to change movement habits that are causing ongoing injuries and compensations, they must recognize the patterns that they developed at the time they were injured. It might seem like common sense that, once we heal, we would start moving in the same pattern that we had before the injury, but that is not necessarily true.

Unless the rehab we undergo after an injury works with the whole system and not only with the area that was injured, the person will continue to move as if the pain and injury are still there. From

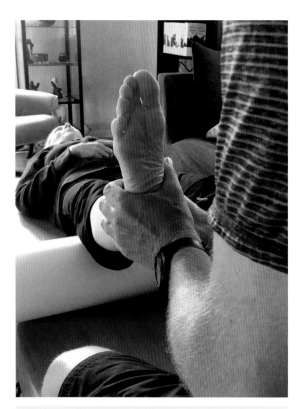

Figure 20.1
Pushing through the sole of the foot.

Courtesy of Staffan Elgelid

a nervous system's perspective that makes sense. Why take a chance and get hurt again? So there are almost always echoes of the injured movement patterns left in us, even after we heal.

After the client did an initial body scan in supine, I started lifting her legs, first the right and then the left, gently pushing on the sole of the foot through the length of the leg so that she could feel compression throughout the lower extremity (Figure 20.1). I experimented with different heights of the leg and angles of hip flexion and abduction until I felt the force go from the sole of the foot through the knee and hip joint, and up through the spine. The purpose of this was to bring awareness to the proprioception in these joints so that the client would more easily feel the difference in weight-bearing while standing. The next step was for her to sense weight-bearing in sitting.

I helped the client to a seated position with the feet on the floor and the knees bent at 90 degrees. I then asked her to sense the weight on her ischial tuberosities (IT) and asked her if she felt equal weight on both ITs. The client had a difficult time sensing her ITs so I asked her to put her hands in between the ITs and the table, thereby increasing the feedback from her own body so that she could feel the difference in weight-bearing between the left and right IT. The client noticed that she put more weight on the left IT. She then weight-shifted left and right until she felt the same pressure under both ITs. Once she could unweight either IT and return to equal weight, it was time for weight shift in standing.

The client moved from sitting to standing and again was asked to sense if she was putting more weight on one side or the other. She felt that she was putting more weight on the left leg but was not sure. Just as I had used the ITs for feedback while sitting, I now introduced the three points of the foot (first and fifth metatarsal head and calcaneus) for feedback in standing. I asked the client to lie down in supine again and put gentle pressure on the above three points in each foot so that she could sense and differentiate them. She then stood up and was asked again to sense whether she was putting more weight on one foot than the other. She now said that she felt more pressure on the three points on the left foot, and that she put more weight on the first metatarsal on the right foot and the fifth metatarsal on the left foot. She then weight shifted on her feet from left to right and from front to back until she felt she had equal weight on the three points on both feet. After that, I asked her to weight shift out of equal weight-bearing to see how quickly she could regain it afterward

Session 2. The stress fractures

In the first session, the focus was on teaching the client to notice unequal weight-bearing, with the attention being on the increased weight being borne on the left side. In the second session, the focus was on the affected right side. Since the initial sprains were on the lateral aspect of the right ankle, the client had protected the ligaments on that side by constantly contracting the peroneal muscles on the outside of the lower leg as a way to avoid pain with movement. Contracting the peroneal muscles influences the mobility of the cuboid bone, lifting it up, and also affects the ability of the fourth and fifth metatarsals to adapt to the ground. The fourth and fifth metatarsals have the most mobility of the metatarsals and, by adapting to the ground on initial contact, are used to lessen the shock of the foot strike. As the foot rolls through the stance phase of the gait, it rolls toward the less mobile first and second metatarsals to get ready for push off.

It was clear that the client had lost the flexibility and adaptability of the fourth and fifth metatarsals and instead landed on the stiffer, medial part of the foot. We worked on the theory that the lack of adaptability of the fourth and fifth metatarsals was one of the causes for the stress fractures in the right foot. To bring back the adaptability of the foot we used an "artificial floor."

With the client in supine I placed a wooden clipboard against the sole of her right foot (Figure 20.2). Initially the board was moved from side to side across the sole of the foot. I then held it more toward the lateral aspect of the foot and maintained the pressure there for about 15 seconds until I felt a softening of the lateral aspect of the foot, including the fourth and fifth metatarsals. This

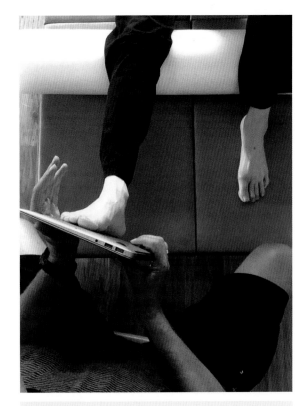

Figure 20.2
Using an "artificial floor."

Courtesy of Staffan Elgelid

was done so that all the tension on the outside of the foot and leg would decrease. To keep stretching out the lateral aspect of the foot would not be congruent with "letting go" for the nervous system. By putting the lateral aspect of the ankle in a shortened/relaxed position, the nervous system could let go of the holding of that aspect of the ankle.

After the nervous system was introduced to a sense of safety, I slowly started moving the clipboard toward the medial side of the foot. By transferring the pressure across, the lateral side slowly re-established its "normal" length. I continued working with the artificial floor, putting the client's foot and ankle in a variety of positions, while paying attention to ensure she did not tighten up the peroneal muscles, thereby avoiding triggering a fear response from her nervous system.

After working with the client in supine, I asked her to move to a seated position with her feet flat on the floor. She was now able to actively perform similar movements to the ones she had passively felt during the artificial floor lesson. That is, she rolled

the sole of the foot from the first to the fifth metatarsal and back again several times. While doing this movement, the client also focused on the position of the knee while rolling the bottom of the foot on the floor.

When rolling the bottom of the foot like this, there is a tendency to let the knee move in the same direction as the foot rolls. I asked the client to ensure this didn't happen. The knee had to be kept still: in the same position as when there was equal pressure on the three points of the foot. The client quickly learned how far she could roll the bottom of the foot before the knee moved. She then reversed that movement and moved the knee from side to side, but without losing the equal pressure on the three points. This differentiation was performed so that the client got a clear sense of the difference between moving the leg with the foot stable on the floor, and moving the foot under a stable leg. When someone sprains an ankle repeatedly, the nervous system becomes too good at protecting the joint and often this differentiation is lost.

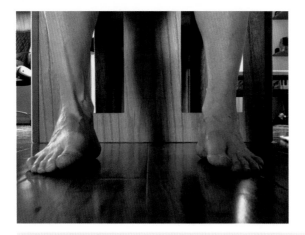 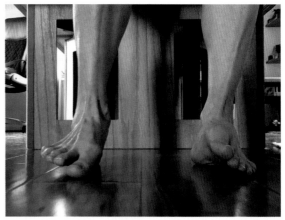

Figure 20.3
(A and B) Differentiating movements of the foot and ankle.

Courtesy of Staffan Elgelid

The client's homework was to do the same kind of foot/ankle movements in sitting with her left foot, and then do the movements in sitting with both feet at the same time but in a variety of combinations (Figure 20.3). That is, she could roll the pressure of the right foot toward the fifth metatarsal and the pressure on the left foot to the first metatarsal or vice-versa. Alternatively, she could roll the pressure on both feet to the fifth or first metatarsal or roll one foot at a faster pace than the other. The homework focused on making the nervous system break up the pattern of stiffness in the feet and for the client's feet to become more "agile," and less injury prone.

Session 3. Agility in standing

The first and second session had focused on weight-bearing throughout the lower extremity and mobility of the bones in the foot. The third lesson reviewed the first two lessons and combined them with the client standing.

This lesson started with the client lying supine. I combined lessons one and two using the artificial floor as a way to heighten her sensation of the three points of each foot (first and fifth metatarsal heads and calcaneus). The big difference was that this time I did not move the artificial floor; instead the client pushed her foot, focusing on creating equal pressure on the three weight-bearing points, while I held the wooden clipboard rigidly. This not only increased her awareness of the three points of the foot, it also created compression into the joints of the lower extremities and the spine, something that we had done passively in lesson one. In lesson one it was me that provided the push to create joint compression; in this lesson, it was the client. The client then pushed and rolled the foot in some of the various combinations used in session two. To involve more of the whole nervous system, though, she also involved movements of the neck and eyes,

sometimes moving in the same directions as the ankle roll and sometimes opposite. I let the client play with some of these movement differentiations between the foot/ankle and neck/eyes. After completing this part of the lesson, making sure that the client could perform these movements in supine, she moved to the standing position.

When standing, the client first found equal weight-bearing of the three points before starting to differentiate between a variety of movements. She began by rolling both feet to the outside, then to the inside; next, the right foot to the outside and the left one to the inside, while maintaining equal weight-bearing on both feet. Following this, she made the same movements, but now with more weight on the front of the feet and then with more weight on the back of the feet. The last differentiation was to do the same again, but with more weight-bearing on the right foot and then the left foot.

By rolling the foot in all these different combinations, the client's nervous system was introduced to a number of possibilities that can occur during daily activities. To only do the rolling movements when in equal weight-bearing does not mirror reality. In real life we cannot control our weight-bearing status during everyday activities or in competition, so we must train the nervous system to recognize all possible variations. To finish up the standing/agility lesson, the client also incorporated the movements of the neck and eyes with the movements of the feet and ankles.

At the end of this third lesson, the client felt satisfied with her progress and ready to return to athletic activities, safe and secure that her nervous system could handle any position that the lower extremities might be in without injuries to her ankles or feet.

Please note that in the above case study, physical therapists had already taken care of strength, flexibility, and balance. My job as a Feldenkrais practitioner was to bring awareness to the client, so she could perceive differences in how she was weight-bearing, appreciate how the whole system was involved and had adapted to her injury, and to give her options in how she used her ankles and feet.

Summary

To summarize, the Feldenkrais Method can help rehab personnel working with clients with orthopedic injuries by following four simple steps:

1 Bring awareness to how clients use themselves at the present time. The way they use themselves is usually dependent on how the nervous system protected them after they got injured.

2 After the person has become aware of how they are using themself in a non-optimal way based on a previous injury, you can start to move the person, passively and then actively, in a way that creates a safe movement for the nervous system. Move slowly and gently so that no red flags go up in it.

3 Start with the person in a supported position on the table, where the nervous system can relax and the person does not have to hold themself up against gravity. This will avoid them using unnecessary muscular holding patterns.

4 Advance the person to seated and standing positions, making sure that they can still perform the movements that were introduced in the non-gravity situation. Here it is important to notice that the person should be able to go into and out of the habitual patterns. It is not a question of removing the habitual patterns, but more about having several different patterns available for the nervous system to choose from.

I almost forgot: number 5 is to make sure you have raised the person's curiosity about movement patterns, so when they go home they will continue to play with the patterns of the previously injured area, as well as in other areas of their body and life. Then they will have gained more than rehabilitation out of the rehab session – they will have had a lesson that can change their life.

Other resources

Bosch, F. 2015. *Strength Training and Coordination: An integrative approach*, translated by Kevin Cook. 2010 Publishers, Rotterdam.

Claxton, G. 2015. *Intelligence in the flesh: Why your mind needs your body more than it thinks.* Yale University Press, New Haven, CT.

Doidge, N. 2007. *The Brain that Changes Itself: Stories of personal triumph from the frontiers of brain science.* Viking Books, New York.

Doidge, N. 2015. *The Brain's Way of Healing: Remarkable discoveries and recoveries from the frontiers of neuroplasticity.* Viking Books, New York.

Epstein, D. 2019. *Range: Why generalists triumph in a specialized world.* Riverhead Books, New York.

Feldenkrais, M. 1990. *Awareness Through Movement.* Harper One, New York.

Hackney, P. 1998. *Making Connections: Total body integration through Bartinieff fundamentals.* Gordon & Breach, Amsterdam.

Hargrove, T.R. 2014. *A Guide to Better Movement: The science and practice of moving with more skill and less pain.* Better Movement, Seattle.

Key, J. 2018. *Freedom to Move: Movement therapy for spinal pain and injuries.* Handspring Publishing, Edinburgh.

Rywerant, Y. 1983. *The Feldenkrais Method: Teaching by handling.* Keats Publishing, New Canaan, CT.

Taylor, M.C. 2019. *Embody the Skeleton: A guide for conscious movement.* Handspring Publishing, Edinburgh.

Ankle Differentiations *Awareness Through Movement* Audio Lesson taught by Staffan Elgelid

Introduction

Many people living with neurological conditions, such as those recovering from a stroke, brain trauma due to an accident, or those affected with a disease such as multiple sclerosis or Parkinson's disease, have found that the Feldenkrais Method has been of great benefit in helping them to live more fully, despite challenges to their ability to move easily. Dr Feldenkrais himself worked with many people with neurological conditions; and the only extended case study he wrote, *Body Awareness as Healing Therapy: The case of Nora* (1977), concerns a woman recovering from a stroke.

I have used the Feldenkrais Method to help hundreds of people with neurological conditions regain movement, recover function, and re-establish a sense of self. For ten years I worked in a neurological rehabilitation unit attached to a major metropolitan public hospital as part of a physiotherapy team. Over the past decade I have continued working with people with different neurological conditions in my Feldenkrais practice, marveling at how this gentle approach can evoke such powerful changes in people's lives.

This chapter will explore the Feldenkrais Method in neurological rehabilitation in terms of neuroplasticity and brain recovery. I also describe how I have used Feldenkrais in my work with clients.

The changing brain

The brain needs three types of systems or processes to be operating for it to function. First, there are the anatomical structures that make up the nervous system. This includes different types of neurons, pathways, tracts, and nuclei that we call the brain. Second, there are the electrical impulses that transmit signals along these neural pathways, bringing the brain to life with a kaleidoscope of constantly changing patterns of firing. Third, there is the chemical "soup" in which the brain is bathed. This mixture of neurotransmitters and other chemicals regulates the amount and types of activity occurring in the brain (Claxton 2015, pp. 80–90). Any damage or disease of the brain has the potential to disrupt one or more of these processes.

When we talk about neurological rehabilitation, which of these systems are we working with? Advances in neuroscience have confirmed that the brain and its neurotransmitters are able to be changed through experience (Doidge 2007). The actual structures of the brain (thickness of the tracts, numbers of synapses, etc.) can change in response to a person's experiences. Specific training regimes – such as practice of a musical instrument – can result in increased mass in certain parts of the brain or improved connectivity between regions of the brain (Doidge 2007). Conversely, deprivation of stimulation from lack of movement and/or sensation can lead to brain shrinkage (Doidge 2007). Through rehabilitation, we are aiming to change the patterns of firing and strength of synaptic connections in the brain, resulting in possible changes to its actual structure over time. There have been some encouraging recent studies that have confirmed that Feldenkrais Method techniques can result in changes to the brain connectivity/activity, as identified on MRI (Verrel et al. 2015).

When thinking about how the brain works, it's useful to know that the brain has a representation of the body literally mapped out on its surface.

There is a sensory map and a motor map. Feldenkrais (1990) had an interest in these brain maps and speculated on how they might be changed, even though he worked before brain imaging. He also postulated that we act according to our self-image (Feldenkrais 1990, p. 3), and therefore the clearer and more accurate that self-image or map, the better will be our movement. We know now that we don't just have sensory and motor maps (Carter 2010), that in fact there are many ways our brains map, or represent, our bodies and the world around us – not just in the cortex, but also in subcortical structures. Indeed, in describing the Feldenkrais Method in his book *The Brain's Way of Healing*, Doidge states, "Slower movement [as used in Feldenkrais Method teaching] leads to more subtle observation and map differentiation, so more change is possible" (Doidge 2015, p. 173).

A Feldenkrais lesson also induces a calm state. Doidge postulates that this may have a neuromodulation effect on the recovering brain, due to the chemicals that are released when a person enters this state (Doidge 2015). This calm and attentive state, which Anat Baniel refers to as having the learning switch turned on (2012), is an important element of the Feldenkrais Method, and it can be particularly beneficial in neurological rehabilitation. Doidge (2015) has described this element of neurological recovery, when the balance of firing patterns within the brain is being restored, as an essential step in brain healing, and one that the Feldenkrais Method can assist in.

Rehabilitation in neurological conditions is therefore all about providing the sort of experiences that optimize recovery, lead to positive changes in the brain's structure and improved connections between neurons, and also help the injured brain to settle into a better condition for recovery.

The sensory system

All experiences that originate outside the body are transmitted to the brain via the sensory systems – through touch, movement, sight, sound, etc. It is through the sensory system that we have the opportunity to reshape the recovering brain. Exercise for a weakened muscle may result in a strengthened muscle, but the very act of trying to perform that exercise is sending enormous quantities of information to the brain. Muscles directly performing the task, for example, receive information from other muscles acting to stabilize the inactive parts, from the joints involved in the movements, from the skin in contact with supporting surfaces as the weight is shifted on that support, from the vestibular system about any movements through space, and from the visual system about the environment in which the action is being performed. There is also the cognitive processing load: trying to achieve a certain goal, trying to do it correctly, being fearful of hurting oneself or falling, taking in feedback from the instructor, and so on. All this information has to be collated within the brain and processed at lightning speed to inform the next movement; it is an endless loop between sensory information arriving and motor commands being sent down to the muscles. Even performing a so-called simple exercise can be overwhelming for a recovering brain. It is therefore vitally important in rehabilitation to provide the brain with information that will be not only beneficial for recovery but easy to process; information that makes sense and has meaning to the brain. This is what the Feldenkrais Method is all about.

Fundamental concepts of the Feldenkrais Method

Dr Feldenkrais was aware of the potential of the brain to change a long time before the term neuroplasticity became an accepted concept. (It did not come into common use in mainstream science until after his death in 1984.) However, he constructed his method on the understanding that information fed into the nervous system will drive change in that system (Feldenkrais 1990), a concept now known as "experience-dependent plasticity." Feldenkrais Method techniques of very specific forms of touch and movement were intended to deliver very specific types of information to a person's nervous system as well as helping them to recover lost function and integrate relearned movements into their preserved movement repertoire.

Feldenkrais understood that there is a constant interplay between part and whole in how we function (i.e., that no part moves in isolation from the whole). Even if only one part is moving, the rest of the body is constantly adjusting to these movements in order to remain stable. He appreciated that we always move within an environment, which means the outside world and gravity always need to be considered in any movement, even if we are not in an upright position. This includes information coming in from our eyes and skin, telling us where we are and what's happening around us.

We move to perform a function, so at the core of every movement there needs to be an intention. Feldenkrais understood that as humans we are born being unable to walk and talk; we *learn* these skills, and *how* we learn these skills can give us insight into how to relearn and improve them. Feldenkrais also understood that we cannot separate thinking, moving, feeling, and sensing. These processes are all happening simultaneously and can be considered "two sides of the same coin" (Claxton 2015), so we cannot affect one without affecting the others.

This richness of understanding, about us as humans acting in our own worlds, is part of what distinguishes the Feldenkrais Method from other rehabilitation approaches, such as physiotherapy.

An "exercise" in the Feldenkrais Method is never just a repeated movement, but rather an exploration, with a rich embrace of variability that makes every movement a learning opportunity (Connors et al. 2010). Every movement in a Feldenkrais lesson is an opportunity for the brain to make countless meaningful connections; the movements are grounded in the relationship with the surrounding environment, the purpose of the action, and an awareness of the self who is performing that movement.

After an injury or damage to our brain, there may be physical changes to the connections within it. One or several areas of the brain may be overactive or underactive. While we cannot physically get into the brain and change connections through the Feldenkrais Method, what we can do is to modify the input and the output from the brain.

Input into the brain

We can modify sensory inputs to the brain by sending them to areas that may not be receiving any input from an area of the body. Lack of input from an area will alter the cortical map of that area, even if there is no damage to that brain region. Doidge (2007) describes studies by Michael Merzenich, a pioneer in neuroplasticity, which found that even after only a few days, sensory maps became diminished and lost specificity if that region of the brain was not receiving input from its usual source.

I was working with a person who had altered sensory awareness of her right foot due to multiple sclerosis. After some very detailed touch and movement work, such as small, precise movements of the ankle, mid-foot, and toes of the right foot, she stood up and exclaimed with delight that she felt like she now had an elephant's foot to stand on! Her awareness of that foot had increased significantly, and with it also her ability to put her weight on it and stand more steadily.

The Feldenkrais Method delivers input to the brain with exquisite precision. As Baniel, one of Feldenkrais' original students, describes, "... the brain's ability to perceive fine differences is at the heart of its ability to generate new information for organizing new, more refined and more exacting action and for overcoming limitations" (Baniel 2012, p. 113). This is one of the distinguishing features of the method. Movements can be very small, and very slow. They can be isolated to one specific area of the body, but always with the whole in mind. This narrow focus directs attention on one small body part, and hence one small part of the brain's body map. The aim is to keep the focus on the primary area, but expand attention gently and gradually to adjacent, and then more distant areas and connections, until the whole is finally illuminated, and the connections between the parts have been clarified.

A whole area may be neglected in a person's self-image, so that until a person "finds" that part of themselves again, their ability to move it will be limited.

Case Study 1

Several years ago I worked with a man who had suffered a massive stroke affecting the right side of his brain. Not only could he not move his left arm and leg, but initially he had lost awareness that the left side of his body even existed. An art therapist and I were collaborating on a research project at the time, investigating the relationship between recovery of function and perceived self-image following a stroke (Connors and Grenough 2004). In the art therapy session, this man drew a series of pictures of himself which dramatically illustrated this damaged self-image as well as the changes that took place over time. In the first picture, he drew himself

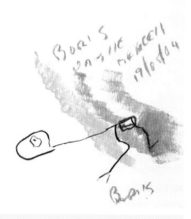

Figure 21.1
Beached.

Courtesy of Karol Connors

with only one arm and leg, washed up on a beach. When prompted by the art therapist, "Is there anything else you'd like to add?" he replied, "Sorry," and added his swimming trunks to the drawing, but not the missing left arm and leg. He thought the image looked complete (Figure 21.1).

Sometime later, he drew himself as standing with two legs, but still somewhat suspended in space, floating, and near the right edge of the page (Figure 21.2). A few weeks later, he had both arms and both legs represented, and I was especially pleased to see that the feet, which we had been

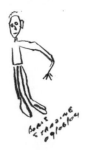

Figure 21.2
Standing.

Courtesy of Karol Connors

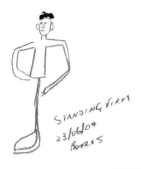

Figure 21.3
Standing firm.

Courtesy of Karol Connors

doing a lot of work on with touch, movement, and weight-bearing, were now evident in the picture, and that he wrote "standing firm" (Figure 21.3). He also drew himself closer to the centre of the page and was clearly feeling differently about himself compared to the first "beached" drawing.

The importance of function

Function is a concept that permeates all of the Feldenkrais Method, and it is equally important in neurological rehabilitation. This is evident from the name which Dr Feldenkrais gave to his hands-on work: *Functional Integration*. Any movement is always considered within the context of the function the person is trying to perform. Mobility in the ankle joint is not considered a goal in the Feldenkrais Method, but the ability to walk over uneven surfaces is. Flexibility in the ribs is not important in itself, but the ability to breathe deeply when needed and turn easily to look behind are core functions for any person. This approach therefore is deeply congruent with rehabilitation, which is all about helping a person regain the ability to function as independently as possible. The underlying intention to use movement to improve functional activity is also one of the features of the work that distinguishes the Feldenkrais Method from other body work approaches or techniques, such as yoga, tai chi, or even Pilates in its original form.

Movement in the field of gravity was a concept that fascinated Dr Feldenkrais, and rehabilitation is indeed fundamentally about getting someone up and out of bed and back into life. One of his earliest books was titled *Body and Mature Behaviour: A study of anxiety, sex, gravitation and learning* (1949), and he continued these themes in his seminal book *Awareness Through Movement*, first published in 1972. I have found the first movement lesson in this later book, describing rising from sitting to standing, to be profoundly useful for many, many people who are relearning the lost skill of standing. He describes subtle concepts involved in this task, such as weight shift over the feet, organization of the flexors and extensors of the thighs and trunk, and the importance of focusing on the task rather than the outcome. He then provides movement exercises to help improve these factors. It is a great example of his understanding of functional movement and the simple but masterful lessons he devised.

Let us consider in more detail how a Feldenkrais practitioner might work with a student experiencing mobility difficulties. It is very common for people with neurological conditions to have problems with mobility. This might be related to motor disturbances (e.g., muscle weakness, spasticity, dystonia, coordination issues, or a combination of all of these), but there may also be issues with diminished, altered, or absent sensation from the lower limbs, such as numbness in the feet or lack of positional sense in the joints.

Lower limb problems after neurological injuries

Very often, following a stroke or head injury, lower limb problems are more pronounced further away from the center of the body. Together with the tendency for a foot to be inverted, there is increased activity in the calf muscles and decreased activity in the muscles at the front of the calf, so that the person walks with a twisted, dropped foot, which is also unstable to stand on.

To start addressing these problems, the Feldenkrais practitioner might start working on the student's feet, with the student comfortably lying on their back, with foam rollers under their knees and ankles to allow easy movements of the hips, knees, and ankles.

The practitioner might start "mapping the territory" on the affected foot, or on both feet depending on the needs of the student. This would involve gently but firmly pressing along the length of the metatarsal bones; individually defining the length, breadth, and width of each toe; outlining the arch of the foot; and pressing onto the ball and heel of the foot.

The pressure would be carefully directed up along the skeleton, creating compression forces up *through* the ankle, knee, hip, and spine, from a myriad of different angles. Each wave of pressure sends information to the central nervous system about the foot, and about the leg. This is a very novel experience for the brain: for the body to be very relaxed so that there are few other competing inputs, and no tasks to perform. Often the student will also close their eyes, so that the entire attention can be focused on the incoming somatosensory information. This allows the student to concentrate fully on sensing parts of themselves in a way that can't happen in an upright dynamic situation when there are so many other competing demands on their neural processing systems. This way of working with the student focused on sensory inputs is one of the unique characteristics of the Feldenkrais Method.

Once the structure of the foot is mapped, the movement landscape is being mapped. Individual, isolated movements will be recognized at first, as the potential of each joint to move, and each muscle to lengthen, is clarified. These isolated movements of individual joints can gradually be linked with whole leg movements: inversion of the ankle, then inversion of the ankle combined with internal rotation of the hip; eversion of the ankle with external rotation at the hip; dorsiflexion of the ankle with a hint of hip/knee flexion added. Part and whole, always dancing between the two, and maintaining the internal image for the student.

Then more complex patterns can be built. For example, ankle inversion with hip external rotation; ankle eversion with hip internal rotation. There can be variations in speed, in amplitude, in the angle of pressure up the skeleton. Variations in the sequencing of which part moves first can be tried. Variations by adjusting the practitioner's hand positions can bring different parts of the foot and leg into focus.

The student may be invited to participate in these movements, depending on their ability, or just to track and pay attention to what differences they can feel.

The legs may then be repositioned into a "standing" position, with the soles of the feet on the table and the knees bent. More movement explorations would be continued in this position, beginning to press the feet into the table and lift the pelvis to discover how the ankles, knees, and hips work synergistically as the student starts to move in the field of gravity.

The student then sits and stands, if possible, to integrate these new movement possibilities into the upright organization of standing and walking. Following this *Functional Integration* lesson, there may be specific movement sequences that the student will be encouraged to explore on their own.

This is a lot of information to process, so frequent short rests or pauses allow the student's brain time to absorb this complex information without being overwhelmed. This concept of frequent rests or pauses is another distinguishing feature of the Feldenkrais Method.

Case Study 2: Carla

Let's meet Carla, a woman recovering from a stroke that affected the right side of her body. Although she has achieved independent walking with the aid of a stick and an ankle orthosis, she has little ability to move her arm. The illustrations show some of the work we have done together.

In Figure 21.4 I am assisting her to slide the palm of her hand along her thigh. This sliding movement is providing the palm of her hand with tactile stimulation; it is receiving very little stimulation in her

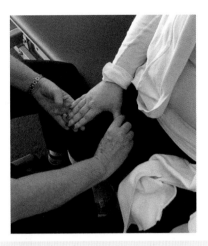

Figure 21.4
Hand on thigh.

Courtesy of Karol Connors

daily life and is therefore at risk of being severely diminished in her brain's sensory map. Simultaneously, she is experiencing synchronized sensations of movement in her wrist, elbow, and shoulder, and she is able to help with these forward and backward sliding movements. Her diminished ability to sense where the hand is in space can be improved by running it along the thigh, as this means she also receives information from that leg about where the hand is, which contributes to helping the brain to track the movements. Another feature of this movement is that by running the hand along the thigh, we are demanding a specific coordination between the elbow and shoulder; to keep the hand in contact with the thigh, the elbow must be extending as the shoulder is flexing. This movement is not only familiar to her – and somewhat comforting – but has the potential to become a movement she can practice herself. We used the hand to explore the outside and inside of the knee in circular movements and also integrated the arm movements with hip flexion and trunk rotation as the hand slid down past her knee to her shin.

Techniques such as sliding a limb over a surface maps out not only the dimensions of that limb through the sensory contact with the surface, simultaneously with proprioceptive input from the muscles and joints informing the brain about changing joint angles and muscle lengths, but the journey through space is also being mapped. All that information needs to be processed simultaneously, hence the need for *slow, precise* movements: to allow a brain that may be processing slowly or is easily overloaded to register and process these inputs.

Reaching is a fundamental activity of the arm, and in Figure 21.5 we are exploring reaching movements out to Carla's right side. We are not only engaging the arm, but also facilitating a weight shift from left to right and practicing forward and side bending in the trunk. This is helping to integrate the less "known" arm with her trunk. Part of the big picture we're also exploring is the space out to this

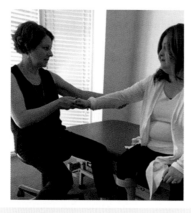

Figure 21.5
Reaching.

Courtesy of Karol Connors

side. Touching the table and sliding her hand on it helps her to "map the territory" of the space around her as well. We can also explore variations in direction, as well as different combinations of rotation of the forearm and upper arm.

To increase the sensory input during these movements, Carla can lean into my resistance or I can push up through the bones of her arm into her shoulder joint and into her trunk, so she senses with her whole body the movements which are being initiated in the arm. This is still an unusual and novel experience for her brain, which consequently will pay full attention to it. It is a functional movement, and we made it meaningful by imagining different items she might be reaching for.

Connecting the known with the unknown is an important part of any learning. We can use this concept to good effect when we place a hand (often in neurological conditions somewhat diminished in the body image) onto the head or face, which is generally still keenly present in the body awareness. For some people this can be quite an emotional connection, and many of my students have cried when they have first had their hand gently placed on their cheek or forehead. There seems to be a sense of relief and comfort in such a familiar gesture. For others, though, it can be disturbing if the hand is so foreign it doesn't register as part of themselves at all. This position can be useful to explore movements such as rolling the head with the hand, as illustrated in Figure 21.6, or turning the hand and head together to elicit turning in the trunk. All the time, we keep in mind how we are engaging the whole of the self and enlarging the image of the self from which we move.

Dr Feldenkrais preferred to talk about improvement rather than recovery when considering neurological rehabilitation, because we cannot recover how the brain was in the past, but there is an endless

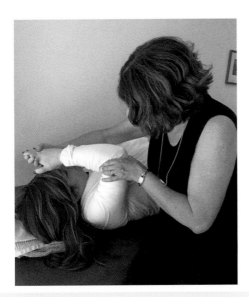

Figure 21.6
Hand to forehead.

Courtesy of Karol Connors

path of improvement that is possible. The Feldenkrais Method has myriad strategies to assist people in following this path.

References

Baniel, A. 2012. *Kids Beyond Limits*. Penguin, New York.

Carter, R. 2010. *Mapping the Mind*. Orion, London.

Claxton, G. 2015. *Intelligence in the flesh: why your mind needs your body more than it thinks*. Yale University Press, New Haven, CT.

Connors, K., Grenough, P. 2004. "Redevelopment of the sense of self following stroke using the Feldenkrais Method," (abstract). Poster presented at the Feldenkrais Annual Research Forum, Seattle WA, August, 2004.

Connors K., Said, C., Galea, M., Remedios, L. 2010. Feldenkrais Method balance classes are based on principles of motor learning and postural control retraining: a qualitative research study. *Physiotherapy* 96:324–336.

Doidge, N. 2007. *The Brain that Changes Itself: Stories of personal triumph from the frontiers of brain science*. Viking Books, New York.

Doidge, N. 2015. *The Brain's Way of Healing: Remarkable discoveries and recoveries from the frontiers of neuroplasticity*. Viking Books, New York.

Feldenkrais, M. 1949. *Body and Mature Behaviour: A study of anxiety, sex, gravitation and learning*. International University Press, New York.

Feldenkrais, M. 1977. *Body Awareness as Healing Therapy: The case of Nora*. Somatic Resources, Berkley, CA.

Feldenkrais, M. 1990. *Awareness Through Movement: Health exercises for personal growth*. Reprint. Harper Collins, New York.

Verrel, J., Almagor, E., Schumann, F., Lindenberger, U., Kühn, S. 2015. Changes in neural resting state activity in primary and higher-order motor areas induced by a short sensorimotor intervention based on the Feldenkrais Method. *Frontiers in Human Neuroscience* 9:232. Available at: http://dx.doi.org/10.3389/fnhum.2015.00232

The Feldenkrais Method of somatic education is a learning process that is useful for managing and reducing chronic pain. This chapter will discuss a conceptual framework combining principles from the Feldenkrais Method and ideas from positive psychology that promote a positive orientation to learning and change for people living with chronic pain.

What is chronic pain?

Chronic pain, also called persistent pain, is a different condition and a different experience from acute pain. Every person has experienced acute pain caused by an injury or illness. We interpret acute pain as danger, and this can motivate us to respond in a way that supports healing or to seek treatment. The expectation is that acute pain will resolve with healing of the injury or appropriate management of the illness. Chronic pain, however, does not go away, and it may vary in intensity and quality throughout the day, a week, or even a lifetime. There may or may not be a specific cause that can be clearly pointed to, and there is no single approach or solution to manage or decrease it. Persistent pain can have a profound and limiting effect on what one does and the way one moves and thinks about oneself. The same sense of danger or threat that is present with acute pain is also present with chronic pain. Chronic pain is a major health condition affecting more than 20 percent of the adults in the United States alone (Dahlhamer et al. 2018).

In 1979, the International Association for the Study of Pain (IASP 2014) defined chronic pain as "an unpleasant sensory and emotional experience associated with actual or potential tissue damage or described in terms of such damage." In reviewing this definition, Cohen, Quintner, and van Ryswick (2018) added: "Pain is a mutually recognizable somatic experience that reflects a person's apprehension of threat to their bodily or existential integrity."

Both definitions speak to the individual nature of the experience of living with chronic pain.

The experience of chronic pain

David Biro, MD, writes in *The Language of Pain: Finding words, compassion, and relief* that the experience of living with chronic pain changes one's perspective. The experience brings a turning inward as the sensations tend to isolate one from the world. The world generally does not know what to do and even turns away from anyone who is suffering (Biro 2010, p. 30). Pain constructs walls between people, and it is nearly impossible to imagine the experience of someone who is in chronic pain. It is important for providers to recognize this separation and to do what they can to demonstrate empathy and compassion toward the person in pain. Effective work with someone with chronic pain requires a holistic orientation and a recognition that the lived experience of chronic pain is real, subjective, and affects all parts of a person's life. It is not enough to think only in terms of improving movement – the person in pain needs to be able to improve their sense of self and the ability to act in the world.

The Feldenkrais Method and positive psychology

The cover of Moshe Feldenkrais' book *Awareness Through Movement* describes it as providing

"Easy to do exercises for improving posture, vision, imagination, and personal awareness," which suggests that there is more to the method than simply improving movement. Feldenkrais expressed the need for self-education, to learn new responses, and to improve how one learns in order to have a more satisfying life. Some of the ideas in the practice of the Feldenkrais Method are also described by Martin Seligman (2012) in *Flourish: A visionary new understanding of happiness and well-being*. For Feldenkrais, the ideas are not abstract concepts to be understood, rather they are ideas that can be made concrete through the experiential process of *Awareness Through Movement*.

For example, Feldenkrais and Seligman both value:

- **Curiosity:** actively engaging in novelty; having a love of learning. The Feldenkrais Method uses the novelty of the movement explorations and the use of a questioning process to evoke a person's curiosity.

- **Open mindedness:** having the ability to change your mind. This is explored through variations in movements such as coordination of the eyes, or breathing, or how different parts of the body are brought into the pattern. In an *Awareness Through Movement* lesson, rather than staying with one solution to a suggested movement exploration, one is asked to experiment.

- **Personal intelligence:** the ability to use one's experience to solve problems. One learns and is asked to use different learning strategies and apply them in the lesson, and later they are available to use in one's life. Strategies such as moving slowly in order to notice how one is performing the movement, shifting attention to different parts of the body, exploring how to make the movement easier, more comfortable

and even aesthetically pleasing are basic to all lessons.

- **Kindness and generosity:** the ability to act kindly and express generosity. One is asked to move without causing pain, and to hold an attitude of kindness toward oneself, being okay with what is possible to do in the present moment; being generous with positive feelings toward oneself.

- **Bravery:** an ability to uncouple fear from the physical response to fear, such as holding the breath or clamping down with the body. This

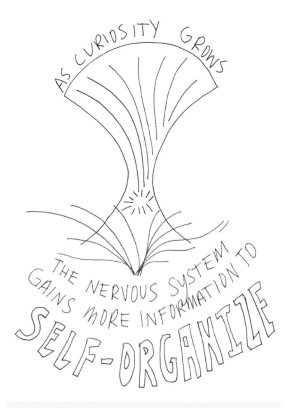

Figure 22.1
As Curiosity Grows.

Courtesy of Tiffany Sankary 2020

is important in order to reduce the fear of movement. Being brave in *Awareness Through Movement* means that one can and will explore what is possible to do, safely, kindly, and with curiosity and an open mind.

These concepts are just a few examples of the links between positive psychology and the Feldenkrais Method. The ideas are woven into an *Awareness Through Movement* lesson and give people a felt sense of what it is like to be open-minded or curious or brave.

The nervous system and chronic pain

Chronic or persistent pain is considered a dysfunction of the nervous system, so improving how it functions will help to reduce such pain. Feldenkrais, in *The Elusive Obvious,* suggests a simple model describing the functions of the nervous system. It's "… important… to understand… the multiple activity of the nervous system. It senses its own body and the objects of the environment and it has curiosity to do these things" (Feldenkrais 2019, p. 129). In this model, curiosity is the driver, stimulating the feedback and perceptual systems into action. As curiosity grows, the nervous system gains more information to self-organize. In the learning processes of the Feldenkrais Method, students are asked to notice, for example, how they are breathing, where contact is made with the floor, how they flex the spine, what differences there are before and after moving, or in the sense of the right and left sides. Questions that explore sensations are valuable to train a person's sensory systems, stimulate curiosity, and help them develop the tools needed to discover what is needed to move comfortably. These kinds of questions redirect the attention away from areas of pain and open the possibility for sensing other aspects of one's experience.

Curiosity and chronic pain

Curiosity can be used to interrupt and change a pain pattern. A healthy person is curious: open to new ideas and possibilities. One of the long-term effects of persistent pain is a diminished sense of curiosity about oneself and/or the world. Often someone with chronic pain has been given rules to follow and told what to do and what not to do by a provider. Following rules coming from expert recommendations, such as "don't move your spine," "never lie on your belly," or "never kneel" do not help, and may result in a sense of hopelessness – a belief that nothing will help and there is nothing one can do to improve.

One of the enduring ideas from the Feldenkrais Method is that one can always improve. Awareness is the most important tool needed for this. Awareness allows one to know what one is doing, its effect, and how to make changes to improve the quality of one's organization.

Feldenkrais lessons direct one's attention to how one is moving, as well as to how one is sensing, feeling, and thinking. This learning methodology asks the student to shift attention away from the urge to succeed and stay in the process of learning. Learning actively restores a healthier function of the nervous system by evoking curiosity. A student discovers new things about themselves, and about how they can change and gain resources for pain management.

Self-imaging and chronic pain

Feldenkrais defines self-image as having four aspects: moving, sensing, feeling, and thinking.

In *Awareness Through Movement, Health exercises for personal growth* the opening sentence is:

We act according to our self-image.

Feldenkrais 1972, p. 3

Each one of us speaks, moves, thinks, and feels in a different way, each according to the image of himself that he has built up over the years. In order to change our mode of action we must change the image of ourselves that we carry within us.

Feldenkrais 1972, p. 10

For Feldenkrais, the concept of self-image includes more than just one's body image. However, body image and self-image are related concepts. According to Rice, Hardenbergh, and Hornyak (1989), three elements are needed to develop a healthy perception of the self:

1 A healthy body image is flexible, with an understanding that the body is fluid and can change.

2 A healthy body image is grounded in the actuality of living in the world.

3 A healthy body image is three-dimensional, is more than how one looks and includes all parts of the self, and movement.

Rice et al. (1989) further state that when the body image is disrupted, the image becomes fixed and there is a lack of a sense of joy.

Lotze and Moseley (2007) investigated how the body image is distorted in people with chronic pain. This distortion includes changes in the neural representations of the body image in the primary sensory and the primary motor cortices of the brain. These neural representations or patterns are changed by one's experiences, becoming stronger with use and with attention, and weaker with inattention and lack of use.

Moving and chronic pain

A person's movement changes as a reaction to injury and pain. There is a natural response that causes a guarding and holding of the muscles to protect one from moving in ways that might cause more damage or re-injury. This is an intelligent and appropriate response initially. However, the limitation of movement can become fixed and continue long after the injury has healed. Over time, one develops restrictions in the body positions and postures and in both the type of movement and amount of movement that can be comfortably done. The movement repertoire shrinks, and fundamental movement relationships, such as that between the head, spine, and pelvis are disrupted. Parts of the body act independently and there is a loss of integration of the whole body.

Some examples of dysfunctional movement patterns commonly seen in people with chronic pain are:

- using more effort than is needed for the task by over-contracting muscles;

- recruitment of muscle groups that are not part of the movement pattern (Feldenkrais [2019, p. 94] describes this as "parasitic action");

- using smaller muscles for big actions;

- using bigger muscles for small actions;

- a lack of appropriate distribution of movement through the whole body, thereby having too much strain or emphasis on a particular joint or joints. There are problems with both the quality of the movement and the quantity.

Dysfunctional movement patterns can take on a compulsive character, become habitual and familiar, and it may seem to the person that there is no other way to move. The effects of poor quality of movement include muscular fatigue, muscle and joint strain or damage, decreased circulation, nerve impingement, digestive and respiratory health issues, increased pain, and more.

In chronic pain, there can be excessive muscular holding and a poor quality of muscular

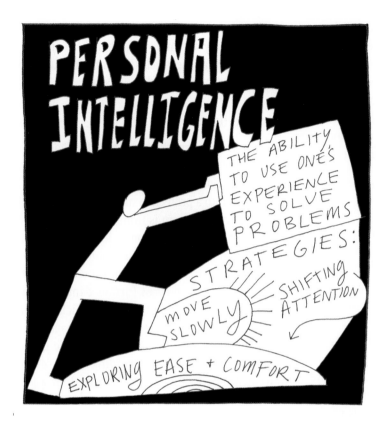

Figure 22.2
Personal Intelligence.

Courtesy of Tiffany Sankary 2020

coordination. Feldenkrais students learn to use the skeleton for support and the muscles for movement. The exploration process of *Awareness Through Movement* lessons directs a student's attention to the movement of the skeleton in space. Students are guided to explore spatial relationships between the joints and body parts, such as length of the sides or spine. There are specific movement explorations focusing on the sense of support through the bones.

Feldenkrais lessons emphasize the quality of movement, such as moving with ease, comfort, and pleasure. Emphasis is also placed on sensing the quality of breathing while moving, and especially on not holding the breath. When a client first begins *Awareness Through Movement* lessons, the range of comfortable movement may be quite

small. Many students with pain report the value of beginning with imagined movements before progressing to small movements as part of regaining ability (Smyth 2018). Gradually, as awareness increases and the confidence in the body is restored, the range of movement is enhanced. Balance, breathing, and coordination improve.

Sensing and chronic pain

For a person with persistent pain, sensing may become focused around its presence or absence. They may lose the nuance and subtlety of other sensations of being alive, especially the pleasant ones. Proprioception is limited because the person is not fully moving all of the joints and muscles in the body. There may be a loss of the ability to interpret sensations, or a lack of sensitivity to them. Feldenkrais lessons direct attention to qualities of sensation (e.g., of contact, skeletal support, resistance, and ease of movement) as well as to the sense of the physical dimensions of the body and how the body and its parts are moving through space. As a result, the student develops greater choices in proprioceptive possibilities and therefore has more choice in how they move.

Thinking and chronic pain

Someone experiencing chronic pain may find their thinking becomes narrowed, with repetitive thoughts revolving around issues of pain, suffering, loss, and limitation. Feldenkrais lessons help improve thinking by engaging the mind to solve novel movement puzzles. Images are used to organize the student's movement: they engage the thinking self and can help to shift attention to the quality of the experience. Students are encouraged to let go of negative thoughts about their body and movement. Some features of the experience of doing Feldenkrais are shared with mindfulness meditation and other types of mindful practices.

Feeling and chronic pain

A person with chronic pain may have a limited range of feelings, but with those such as depression, fear, a sense of isolation, and lack of hope becoming more predominant. Feelings are associated with a bodily organization. If one changes the body, the mind will change, too. As a person becomes more comfortable and finds new possibilities for movement emerging, there is a shift toward a more positive affect, including hopefulness, joy, and calmness.

Feldenkrais lessons expand a person's repertoire in feelings, sensations, thoughts, and movement, which results in a shift in self-image. People often report not only an improvement in what they can do but also that they feel differently about themselves, including feeling pleasure again.

Pain and danger

Butler and Moseley (2013) in *Explain Pain* bring forward the relationship of pain and danger. The normal reaction to danger is to organize the nervous system into a protective survival response. This is useful when the pain is from an acute injury but not when the pain has become chronic. For example, with an acute injury like a joint dislocation, there is strong pain and it is healthy to limit the joint movement to prevent further damage to the tissues and allow healing to occur. In such an injury, the relationship between tissue damage, pain, danger, and the need for protective muscle guarding is clear. However, these guarding responses and movement restrictions, when continued for a long time, may themselves become the problem and contribute to the development of chronic pain conditions. Chronic pain may result in a fearful orientation to movement: *kinesiophobia*.

Kinesiophobia

Luque-Suarez, Martinez-Calderon, and Falla (2019), in a systematic review, examined 64 research papers on the role of kinesiophobia for people with chronic pain. They found strong evidence that higher degrees of kinesiophobia were related to higher levels of pain, more disability from pain, and a lower quality of life. They noted the importance of assessing and considering a person's fear of movement.

The learning environment in the Feldenkrais Method is intentionally structured to be safe for all levels of movers. The atmosphere is noncompetitive and nonjudgmental. Students are supported and encouraged to move within their own comfort zone, to make their own choices as to how many repetitions to do and when to rest. As persistent pain can make one feel under constant threat, it is imperative that students are not under any pressure and feel safe to explore what they can do without causing additional pain. The emphasis is on discovery and exploration, attending to the quality of one's movement, and observing one's internal process while moving. The student learns to notice what they are doing, how they are doing it, attitudes toward the body and the feelings that rise with changes in movement. Through this process, a student develops new ways to move and, more importantly, gains insight into habits of thinking, sensing and feeling, and, of course, moving. The goal is to learn how to learn, not to please the teacher or match an external arbitrary standard of movement.

Self-organization

"The critical variable of a living system… is its self-organization, which determines both the identity and general configuration (structure) of the system," according to a paper by Cohen, Quintner, and van Rysewyk (2018, p. 2) in which they also noted that this structure is continually being modified as the system adapts to its ever-changing environment.

Self-organization could be described as the ability to adapt to constant changes in one's body and environment. People with persistent pain will benefit from questioning their reaction to interpreting pain as proof of tissue damage. Exacerbations of pain, as in a "flare up," could be due to tissue damage; however, there are many other factors that influence the experience of pain. There is more to it than just having a body that hurts.

Difficulties and distortion in self-organizing alters one's self-image, which results in behavioral

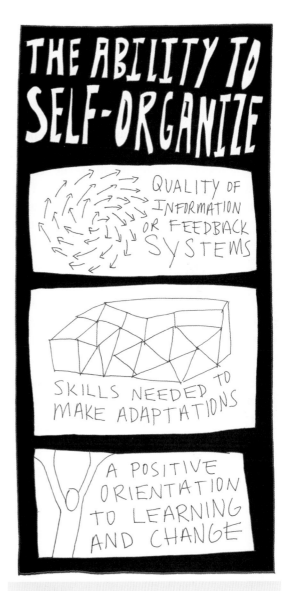

Figure 22.3
The Ability to Self-Organize.

Courtesy of Tiffany Sankary 2020

change. The ability to self-organize depends on several factors including:

- the quality of the information or feedback systems;

- the skills needed to make the adaptations and changes that are needed in the moment;

- a positive orientation toward learning and change.

Persistent pain disrupts and changes the amount and type of feedback that is available to the nervous system. This distortion in feedback processes affects the quality of self-organization. The nervous system is reliant on the continuous feedback from multiple systems and mechanisms for information such as: joint positions, spatial orientation, pressure on parts of the body, or the amount of muscular tension and breathing.

Coordination and control of movement depends on accurate information and the quality of complex feedback loops. Importantly for movement, proprioceptive and kinesthetic senses provide information both unconsciously and consciously.

The kinesthetic sense includes the sense of motion, the position of the joints, the actions of parts of the body, and one's balance. This sense of the body is essential for skillful and comfortable movement, and the Feldenkrais Method uses curiosity to train, develop, and enhance it. Learning to move well and sense oneself while moving is a skill that can be improved. Some of the learning strategies to do so include:

- an emphasis on using curiosity to observe one's habits of moving, thinking, sensing, and feeling, and to do this without judgment;

- focusing on different parts of the moving body;

- changing the focus of attention, for example, to the pressure felt on the floor, or the trajectory of the moving part;

- noticing the effect of the movement on the whole self;

- observing the quality of movement and learning to move with ease and comfort to reduce the sense of effort;

- imagining the movement;

- moving without increasing pain;

- moving while breathing continuously;

- shifting one's attention to different parts of the body while moving;

- using brief rests and pauses to allow one to notice changes.

Both modes of the method – *Functional Integration* and *Awareness Through Movement* – improve one's kinesthetic ability. One can sense more than what hurts. Body awareness improves, and one discovers that there are more options for the way one acts and moves. *Awareness Through Movement* lessons are not only explorations in self-organizing but training to develop the skills to do so. This skill carries over into one's daily life so that one learns to solve such movement problems as sweeping, carrying a baby, or sitting comfortably.

Empowering one's sense of agency

The Feldenkrais Method promotes a sense of agency. Gaining a sense of control over one's body is essential for learning new movement patterns, which in turn lead to improved self-organization. One finds that there are more choices for using one's perceptual abilities and learns how to shift attention from what one cannot do to what one can do. Students learn how to:

- "listen" to their body to better sense the early signs of pain and immediately change how they are moving;

- find and use comfortable positions for rest and tasks;

- use awareness of breathing to guide the sense of comfort and ease;

- direct attention to how all parts of the body participate in any activity;

- overcome movement restrictions by increasing skill, not by forcing or pushing.

Chronic pain is a complex condition and requires a multidimensional systems approach for management. The Feldenkrais Method has tools that are especially relevant for people with chronic pain, and the values embedded within it will support continued personal growth and the skills needed to move toward happiness and well-being. The method stresses learning how to move well, comfortably, and without causing harm to oneself.

References

Biro, D. 2010. *The Language of Pain: Finding words, compassion, and relief.* W.W. Norton, New York.

Butler, D.S., Moseley, G.L. 2013. *Explain Pain*, 2nd edn. Noigroup Publications, Adelaide.

Cohen, M., Quintner, J., van Rysewyk, S. 2018. Reconsidering the International Association for the Study of Pain definition of pain. *Pain Reports* 3(2):e634.

Dahlhamer, J., Lucas, J., Zelaya, C., Nahin, R., Mackey, S., DeBar, L., Kerns, R., Von Korff, M., Porter, L., Helmick, C. 2018. Prevalence of chronic pain and high-impact chronic pain among adults – United States, 2016. *Morbidity and Mortality Weekly Report* 67(36):1001–1006. doi: 10.15585/mmwr.mm6736a2

Feldenkrais, M. 1972. *Awareness Through Movement: Health exercises for personal growth.* Harper & Row, New York.

Feldenkrais, M. 2019. *The Elusive Obvious*, Reprint. North Atlantic Books/Somatic Resources, Berkeley, CA.

IASP (International Association for the Study of Pain) 2014. "ASP Terminology: Pain Terms: Pain,"

https://www.iasp-pain.org/Education/Content. aspx?ItemNumber=1698

Lotze, M., Moseley, G.L. 2007. Role of distorted body image in pain. *Current Rheumatology Reports* 9:488–496. https://doi.org/10.1007/s11926-007-0079-x

Luque-Suarez, A., Martinez-Calderon, J., Falla, D. 2019. Role of kinesiophobia on pain, disability and quality of life in people suffering from chronic musculoskeletal pain: A systematic review. *British Journal of Sports Medicine* 53:554–559.

Rice, J.B., Hardenbergh, M., Hornyak, L.M. 1989. Disturbed body image in anorexia nervosa: Dance/movement therapy interventions. In: L.M. Hornyak and E. Baker (eds.) *Experiential Therapies for Eating Disorders*, pp. 252–278. Guilford Press, New York.

Seligman, M.E. 2012. *Flourish: A visionary new understanding of happiness and well-being.* Simon and Schuster, New York.

Smyth, C. 2018. "The Lived Experience of the Feldenkrais Method PhD." ProQuest Publication number: 13857460, Saybrook University, Oakland, CA. https://pqdtopen. proquest.com/doc/2269043436.html?FMT=ABS

Other resources

Bowes, D. 2008. Feldenkrais Method and Chronic Pain. In: G. Herman and M. French (eds.) *Pain Connection: Making the invisible visible*, pp. 196–199. US Pain Foundation, Tucson, AZ.

Lorig, K.R., Halsted, R., Holman, M.D. 2003. Self-management education: History, definition, outcomes, and mechanisms. *Annals of Behavioral Medicine* 26(1): 1–7. https://doi.org/10.1207/S15324796ABM2601_01

Wyszynski, M. 2010. The Feldenkrais Method for people with chronic pain. *Pain Practitioner* 20(1):56–61.

An easy *Awareness Through Movement* Audio Lesson taught by Deborah Bowes

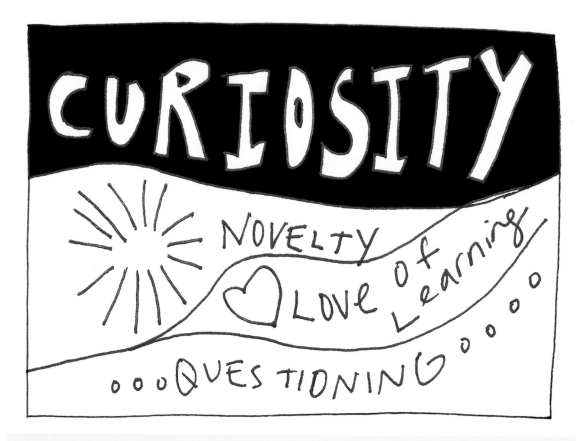

Figure 22.4
Curiosity.

Courtesy of Tiffany Sankary 2020

In this chapter I would like to point to some of the phenomena intrinsic to the Feldenkrais Method that contribute to human development and maturity. People reading Moshe Feldenkrais' books for the first time are often surprised to discover not only movement practices but a mixture of philosophy, psychology, and social critiques in his writings, even as he connects his ideas to the anatomy, physiology, and physics of human action.

Movement and the sense of self are inextricably linked. Through this awareness, and the practices that lead to it, people can: achieve greater autonomy; increase self-efficacy and self-determination; experience self-learning; develop greater authenticity and increased spontaneity; develop greater competence and the feelings of competence; and enhance their capacity for expression. They develop a sense of *I can* (Alon 1996; Sheets-Johnstone 2011; Smyth 2018).

This is the elusively obvious basis of the Feldenkrais Method that puzzles people when they first encounter it. How could a little movement, along with awareness of it, alter my relationship with myself, enhance my effectiveness and creativity, and improve my movement? The genius of the Feldenkrais Method is the process by which it enriches and brings forth moving-sensing bodily experience for the student, and links that to the student's sense of self and *feelings of being* (Ratcliffe 2008).

I argue that various aspects of the Feldenkrais Method practice operate as kinds of "values in action" that can guide how we are in the world. At the same time, these phenomena may operate as deeply lived, bodily metaphors (such as support, balance, integration) that connect the experience of

movement with important aspects of human development. This chapter will necessarily only touch on key points of these phenomena to indicate the chain of experience that shapes our individual moving self.

Maturity

As with other Western somatic thinkers, Feldenkrais developed his method partly in response to the Europe of the early twentieth century. Witnessing the two world wars, the development of conformist mass thought and behavior, and the consequent horrors, encouraged him to look for ways in which people could develop autonomy and authenticity grounded in their own experience, and not through received norms and ideas. Feldenkrais was particularly concerned with how fear and anxiety, especially during development, distorted human development and our options for effective action.

Feldenkrais wrote, "What I understand by maturity, is the capacity of the individual to break up total situations of previous experience into parts and to reform them into patterns most suitable for present circumstances" (2002, p. 196). "Our aim being to further development toward mature adult behavior we are primarily interested in the... acquired responses which are amenable to change" (2002, p. 74). That is, choice about how one is in one's life, and how one responds to one's world, and working with our learned responses in order to change.

The capacity for movement, and sensing oneself through movement, is the ground for improving the sense of self and how we perceive what our world affords us. The Feldenkrais Method involves observing oneself in movement and developing awareness of experiences that occur in various kinds of preconsciously felt experience, as well as consciously identified experience (Legrand 2011, pp. 204–227).

What goes wrong?

First, however, we need to ask: what goes wrong with learning the ability to sense ourselves and to positively alter our own bodily experience? It is hard to develop a positive body image when one's body is the site of oppression and exclusion, and many people are subject to emotional and physical exploitation. A history of the control of others via control of their bodies runs through feudalism, as well as through colonialism and slavery (which together are the basis of systematic racism). In addition, the fear and suppression of sexuality, women's bodies, gender queer and gender non-conforming persons, are also part of the story of the loss of "the bodily." The bodily experience of the oppressed is of little interest to the dominant culture: the experience of one's bodily self as controlled and dominated distorts one's own sense of self.

We are aware of the effects of trauma and its pervasiveness – such as childhood neglect or abuse, sexual assault, and the traumas associated with natural disasters, accidents, and political violence. A large number of modern medical procedures are lifesaving but can be deeply painful or frightening.

All cultures, religions, and families also influence or dictate the kind of movement repertoires and bodily departments allowed for groups of people in society, including and perhaps especially those who critical theory would suggest are considered "other" by the dominant culture, such as girls and young women, and LGBTQ people.

Fear of being unable to support himself was a fear Feldenkrais faced in his youth and contributed to his development of the method. What we do for much of our lives influences what we are able to do. For example, if the shoulders are only used to direct the hands to a keyboard, this diminishes the enormous potential of the human shoulder – and the rest of the body.

Other fears can arise from the experience of illness and injury. Pain is often associated with the fear of movement – kinesiophobia (see Chapter 22). In addition, the fear of social rejection and the inability to find loving and caring relationships drives much of human behavior. It makes evolutionary sense that the part of the brain associated with processing physical pain also becomes activated with the fear of social rejection. Finally, corporations increasingly make use of financial and emotional insecurity to demand greater levels of work output and emotional labor in supporting the goals of the work team and profitability and the company, both of which are major factors in the phenomenon of burnout.

Addressing these aspects of contemporary life are an important part of the potential of the Feldenkrais Method to contribute to health and well-being.

Where to start?

Feldenkrais in *Body and Mature Behavior* wrote of the emotional disturbances associated with trauma, which are the source of the "faulty use of oneself" (2002, p. 20). We feel our emotions in our bodies. In addition to the named emotions, the idea of *affects* also includes mood (as longer-term, perhaps less intense, emotional states), as well as our overall disposition, our patterns, and habits of feelings (Colombetti 2014). Various affects are the basis of emotions or emotional appraisals and show up in qualities of movement (Stern 2010). We can also think about "thinking" as a bodily based function that can be improved through enhancing movement and perception. Our thinking is supported by the body in the present moment and in the patterns learned throughout our lives (Feldenkrais 2019). All these play a part in the movement toward maturity.

Mind-body practices include many that involve stilling the body to still the mind and promote deep physical relaxation. All are useful. At the same time Feldenkrais suggested that, "The aim is not complete relaxation, but healthy, powerful, easy and pleasurable exertion" (2010a, p. 37). The question asked by Feldenkrais, which remains relevant, is how can people achieve and maintain healthy and mature responses to stressors while moving through their lives?

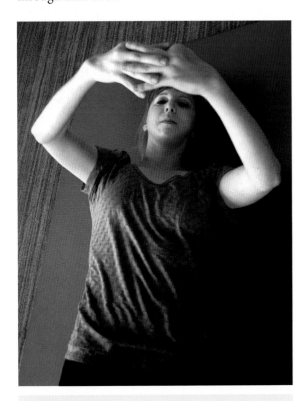

Figure 23.1
Interlacing hands non-habitually.

Courtesy of Cliff Smyth

Feldenkrais (1990) chose the *action system* of sensing and moving as the basis of his method, believing it gave the possibility for effectively and quickly changing our action patterns in the moment, our habits over time, and ultimately our possibilities and potential as humans. Through the movement "doorway," overall patterns of our being can be accessed.

The non-triviality of muscular habits

The Feldenkrais Method focuses on changing the habits of muscular activity to change our movement and our sense of our bodily selves: especially those of excess, parasitic, or misplaced muscular effort. This unnecessary and misdirected high muscular tonus may be global or localized and is often not recognized by the individual. Whatmore and Kohli (1974) used the term *dysponesis* to describe patterns of holding and bracing associated with anticipated actions and acts of perception and thought, which is reflected in many psychophysical conditions such as unexplained headaches and bodily pains, anxiety, and insomnia.

These patterns are closely related to Feldenkrais' idea of how our bodily organization arises and can be distorted in our bodily histories. Feldenkrais (2002) proposes that it is possible to learn a greater sense of poise, less affected by our old patterns of reactivity, that can lead to *acture*: a bodily organization of alert readiness that does not require any preparatory movement or adjustment to move smoothly into action.

Learning to make new and effective responses can be developed through learning to embody certain somatic values in action. The term *values in action*, coined by the founder of positive psychology, Martin Seligman, encompasses a range of values which one may enact in one's life, such as "the love of learning" or "the ability to love and be loved" (2004). Values in

199

action are not static but can be adopted and strengthened. They have the characteristics of *competencies*; that is, they involve skills, values, and abilities we manifest in our action in the world (Boni and Lozano 2007, pp. 819–831). In the Feldenkrais Method, people experience core ideas in action. Here, I am bringing the idea of values in action into the somatic realm: where values in action can be learned, enhanced, and embodied through the process of learning.

Somatic values in action learned through Feldenkrais practice

Here are just some of the somatic values in action that may be developed by practicing the Feldenkrais Method, especially in *Awareness Through Movement*.

- **Slowing (and not hurrying):** an ability to make use of slowing down one's movement to better sense its qualities; to enhance learning; to detect the internal felt sense of hurrying and the senses of acceleration, compression, and distress that come from it; and to find ways to reduce the felt sense of hurrying.

- **Easing (or not efforting):** understanding the value of reducing effort to better sense the qualities of one's movement; to enhance learning; to discover an ability to detect what level of effort is being used and whether it is suitable for the task at hand, thus reducing fatigue and injury; and to develop a sense of the appropriate use of self.

- **Attending:** an ability to direct, focus, and diffuse attention in ways that are appropriate to one's intentions and situation.

- **Breathing:** flexibility in the use of one's breathing apparatus, and an ability to breathe appropriately for the task and situation (for example, to breathe in a rhythm with movement, or to breathe continuously regardless

of the action being performed), generating a sense of being able to "breathe easy."

- **Non-judging:** an ability to attend directly and nonjudgmentally to one's body and movement, thus promoting self-acceptance, self-reliance, and confidence.

- **Not limiting:** understanding the value of not moving to one's physical "limit" in a learning situation but, instead, to create feelings of ease and limitlessness.

- **Supporting:** an ability to find a sense of effectively supporting oneself through the body, especially through the use of the skeleton and breath.

- **Expanding and opening:** an ability to evoke senses of lengthening and widening through movement with attention, and thus promoting a sense of spaciousness and opening to experience.

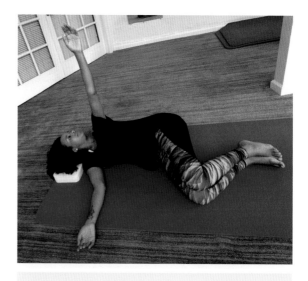

Figure 23.2
Expanding and opening.

Courtesy of Cliff Smyth

- **Balancing**: an ability to find one's balance in gravity and space, use one's body in balanced ways, and evoke a sense of emotional balance in one's life.

- **Integrating**: an ability to integrate parts of the body with each other and the whole body in movement, along with the ability to integrate perception and movement, as well as intention and action in the world.

- **Resting**: an ability to sense the need to rest, and resting when needed, valuing one's own capacities and needs, and attending to the healthy cycles of body and life.

All these contribute to two more somatic values in action which utilize and integrate the previous ones.

- **Self-healing**: an ability to mobilize oneself in ways that promote resilience and allow for effective responses to injury and illness.

- **Self-caring**: developing a caring attitude toward oneself, which one is able to enact through the use of Feldenkrais principles, strategies, and practices, and which can be utilized throughout life.

Aspects of human development

The experience of these and similar values in action provides a basis for experiencing oneself and acting in new ways: for self-directed human development. They allow for greater present-moment awareness, or mindfulness, which can reduce rumination and anxiety. Effective action in the world does not require being continuously aware; however, the process of learning in the Feldenkrais Method requires that attention and awareness be brought to bear during the learning process. This capacity for self-observation in action is a basis of what psychologists have termed *meta-cognition*. The ability to perceive one's own mental and bodily processes allows one

to develop a perspective from which one is able to choose to change one's behavior. From the concrete experience of caring for themselves in Feldenkrais classes, students often adopt a less aggressive, more compassionate attitude toward themselves. It also takes courage to sense one's body – especially if one has a history of trauma, chronic pain or poor body image. Beringer (2010, pp. 33–38) elaborates on Feldenkrais' idea of the self-image, suggesting that this should really be considered as an active and creative process, *self-imaging*; and rather than conceiving of the self as a static thing with fixed characteristics, one should think about the self as a process of *self-ing*.

In Feldenkrais practice the locus of control for learning is with the student. This process of learning how to learn in the Feldenkrais Method is very similar to the process of *self-teaching* as described by philosopher of mind Ryle (1979), who argues that genuine thinking is really a process of experimenting with possible questions and possible solutions, trying on options, and finding solutions that work for the individual.

Finding *how* to do things in ways that are more pleasurable or satisfying may help to shift one's motivations toward greater "intrinsic motivation" (Deci and Ryan 2008, pp. 182–185). Discovering habitual patterns of holding, stuckness, depression, anxiety, or compulsive agreeableness, along with ways to shift them, can "take the brake off" possibilities for more spontaneous responses, toward a greater range of expression and joy in life (Alon 1996).

The experience of *I can*: self-efficacy, competence, and confidence

Feldenkrais *Awareness Through Movement* lessons can be seen as promoting "self-efficacy" (Bandura 1977, pp. 191–215). In other words, there is enough challenge in the learning task for a person to feel that they are really learning or achieving something, and at the same time there is not so much challenge as to cause failure or a sense of being overwhelmed by the task. *Awareness Through Movement* lessons are structured in their movement tasks in sequencing, and framed by the teacher as not having specific goals in terms of the size or shape of the movement, but only goals in terms of the values in action of non-judging, slowing, easing, not limiting, and self-caring.

Taken together, these capacities, learned through the Feldenkrais Method, contribute to a sense of *I can*. The experience of this sense is fundamental to human life: the ability to do and to move in the broadest sense used here, rather than abstracted thinking in words or images, is required to be human and have a world (Sheets-Johnstone 2011). Feldenkrais stated, "Movement is life" (2010b, p. 179). This might be read as a *biological* imperative, but I believe it is also a statement about the *experience* of human life.

Returning to maturity

Feldenkrais saw his method as fostering "the process of self-direction," contributing to maturity through

a greater ability to make distinctions, and based on those distinctions, to make choices (2019, p. 110). Choices become more context-sensitive, effective and coherent, and consistent with our intentions. That experience of choice, of how to respond and how to be, are, in Feldenkrais terms, the basis of maturity. One develops the capacity not just to react to the changing and challenging circumstances of life, but to make an appropriate response. While making distinctions in movement might seem particularly concrete and trivial, the discussion here shows how all distinctions help move us toward greater capacity, caring, competence, and confidence. This provides a basis for positive self-assertion (Alon 1996).

Developing greater awareness enables us to encounter situations, even ones that have similar features of difficulties and trauma that we have previously encountered, and instead of reacting habitually, have the capacity to respond in new, healthy

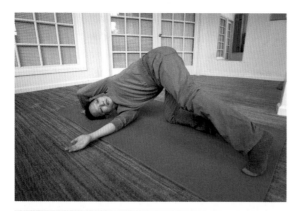

Figure 23.3
Points of support from the ground.

Courtesy of Cliff Smyth

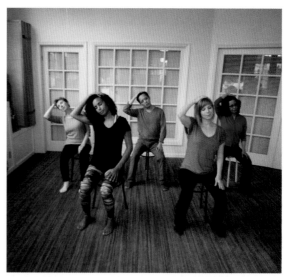

Figure 23.4
Seated *Awareness Through Movement* lesson.

Courtesy of Cliff Smyth

ways consistent with our values and life intentions. That is maturity.

Self-knowledge is a vital part of how we form and carry out our intentions. It is an essential part of our effectiveness; and our ethics. As the body is the site of much of our experience of oppression, it also offers the possibility for finding greater liberation.

At the same time as promoting the process of self-education, Feldenkrais emphasized that choice should not put one in unnecessary conflict with one's environment:

To be of practical use, the mode of doing must not be an ideal, but expedient – one that can be normally used in our present-day society. It is useless to aspire to an idea of being better than everyone else. The main object is to form an attitude and a new set of responses that permit an even and poised application of oneself to the business of living and not create new terrain for conflict. Moreover, the new mode of action must perforce be adjusted to the present environment – even though everybody agrees that our social structure and education need radical improvement if they are to become suitable for a society of creative, evolving, mature adults.

Feldenkrais 2002, p. 107

It is true that it is a mature choice not to engage in *unnecessary* conflict with things as they are. However, with the return to authoritarianism in the West, grounded in racism, sexism, and the denial of human rights, there is an argument that we are returning to the kinds of social conditions that contributed to Feldenkrais' original development of his method. In other parts of the world, old forms of oppression continue and are being updated. New forms of disembodiment and social control, in the form of new technologies, along with the climate emergency, require us all to ask ourselves how we will respond.

It is possible for us to take the awareness of our bodily experience and apply our new skills acquired through practices like the Feldenkrais Method to break down existing situations and generate new ways of responding. Autonomy is not individualism but a capacity for connection with self, and therefore with others. We can use our authentic self-knowledge and self-compassion to connect with others skillfully and compassionately. How will we use the competencies we gain from practices like the Feldenkrais Method to respond to new situations?

References

Alon, R. 1996. *Mindful Spontaneity: Returning to natural movement.* North Atlantic Books, Somatic Resources, Berkeley, CA.

Bandura, A. 1977. Self-efficacy: Toward a unifying theory of behavioral change. *Psychological Review* 84(2):191–215.

Beringer, E. 2010. Self-imaging. *The Feldenkrais Journal* 13.

Boni, A., Lozano, J.F. 2007. The generic competences: An opportunity for ethical learning in the European convergence in higher education. *Higher Education* 54:819–831. https://doi.org/10.1007/s10734-006-9026-4

Colombetti, G. 2014. *The Feeling Body: Affective science meets the enactive mind.* The MIT Press, Cambridge, MA.

Deci, E.L., Ryan, R.M. 2008. Self-determination theory: A macrotheory of human motivation, development, and health. *Canadian Psychology/Psychologie Canadienne* 49(3):182–185.

Feldenkrais, M. (1972) 1990. *Awareness Through Movement: Health exercises for personal growth.* Harper & Row, New York.

Feldenkrais, M. 1998. *The Potent Self: A study of spontaneity and compulsion introduction: love thyself as thy neighbor,* Reprint. Frog Limited & Somatic Resources, Berkeley, CA.

Feldenkrais, M. 2002. *Body and Mature Behavior: A study of gravitation, anxiety, sex and learning.* Frog Ltd/Somatic Resources, Berkeley, CA.

Feldenkrais, M. 2010a. Mind and body. In: E. Beringer (ed.) *Embodied Wisdom: The collected papers of Moshe Feldenkrais,* pp. 27–44. North Atlantic Books, Berkeley, CA.

Feldenkrais, M. 2010b. Movement and the mind, interview with Will Schutz. In: E. Beringer (ed.) *Embodied Wisdom: The collected papers of Moshe Feldenkrais*, pp. 179–189. North Atlantic Books, Berkeley, CA.

Feldenkrais, M. (1981) 2019. *The Elusive Obvious*, Reprint. North Atlantic Books/Somatic Resources, San Francisco.

Legrand, D. 2011. Phenomenological dimensions of bodily self–consciousness. In: S. Gallagher (ed.) *The Oxford Handbook of the Self*. Oxford University Press, Oxford.

Ratcliffe, M. 2008. *Feelings of Being: Phenomenology, psychiatry and the sense of reality*. Oxford University Press, Oxford.

Ryle, G. 1979. *On Thinking*. Rowman & Littlefield, Totowa, NJ.

Seligman, M.E. 2004. *Authentic Happiness: Using the new positive psychology to realize your potential for lasting fulfillment*. Simon and Schuster, New York.

Sheets-Johnstone, M. 2011. *The primacy of movement*, 2nd edn. John Benjamins, Amsterdam.

Smyth, C. 2018. *The Lived Experience of the Feldenkrais Method*. ProQuest Publication number: 13857460, Saybrook University, Oakland, CA. https://pqdtopen. proquest.com/doc/2269043436.html?FMT=ABS [Accessed October 2020].

Stern, D.N. 2010. *Forms of Vitality: Exploring dynamic experience in psychology, the arts, psychotherapy, and development*. Oxford University Press, Oxford.

Whatmore, G.B., Kohli, D.R. 1974. *The Physiopathology and Treatment of Functional Disorders: Including anxiety states and depression and the role of biofeedback training*. Grune & Stratton, New York.

Sliding and Lifting Arm on the Side
Awareness Through Movement Audio
Lesson taught by Cliff Smyth

"There are no limits to our improvement."

Moshe Feldenkrais

How will the Feldenkrais Method continue to survive and thrive, and what are the tests of its longevity? Perhaps the timing is exactly right for the method. Moshe Feldenkrais' work was born under the upheaval of World War II and the need to learn how to survive under conditions of hardship, fighting, and danger.

The personal and economic upheaval for millions of people during the 2020 worldwide pandemic reminded many of wartime situations, when usual routines and structures dissolve and individuals find themselves searching for new pathways. The constraints of sheltering at home and social distancing meant that some looked inward while others sought something new and different. This led to the method's reach being exponentially increased as Feldenkrais practitioners the world over began to teach online – *Awareness Through Movement* classes, workshops, summits, and symposia became abundant. I decided to ask diverse people in the Feldenkrais community what they thought about the future viability of the method.

The Feldenkrais Legacy Forum, a body of Feldenkrais trainers, assistant trainers, and practitioners who are working to ensure that the Feldenkrais Method has a robust future, offered the following statement:

"In the past 50 years, the Feldenkrais Method has grown from the ingenious visions and teachings of one man to the founding basis of a profession. The Feldenkrais Guild® of North America, which

certifies practitioners, has established standards of practice, a code of ethics, and service marks to protect the quality and integrity of the work. It has an active Board of Directors, a Training Advisory Board and is part of the International Feldenkrais Federation, as well as other accrediting organizations around the world.

As with any growing organization, the Feldenkrais profession faces challenges. These arise out of the success and growth of the work and deal primarily with how the organization will provide continuity for the education of new practitioners and their teachers. There is a growing demand for Feldenkrais practitioners, and therefore a need for increasing the number of high-quality educators who will shepherd and mentor future generations.

The Feldenkrais Legacy Forum is working towards including the expertise of the entire practitioner community to create a richer vision of the future which includes a variety of training models. This will ensure that skilled and competent people will continue to teach and provide services to the public. We are confident that the Feldenkrais Method will continue growing a vibrant and dynamic profession."

John Tarr, a Feldenkrais practitioner and assistant trainer working in Sweden, has this perspective:

"Dr Moshe Feldenkrais developed his Method hoping that it would ultimately change humanity for the better. He gave us a way to inquire into ourselves and discover how we act in, and react to, the world around us, based on our personal habits and histories. He also gave us a way of refining our actions, if we so choose, to become more mature and capable humans. During his lifetime, his work was

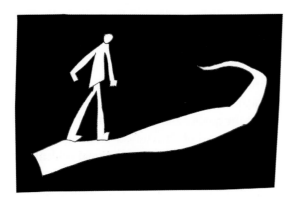

Figure 24.1
On the Path.

Courtesy of Tiffany Sankary 2014. *Feldenkrais Illustrated: The Art of Learning*, Movement and Creativity Press

constantly evolving, leaving me to wonder how it might look now, more than 35 years after his death.

Examining that question has led me to reflect on two seemingly paradoxical statements made by the founder. Dr Feldenkrais said that if he died and came back 30 years later, he hoped that he wouldn't be able to recognize his own Method. He also said that as more and more people discovered how the human nervous system functions, so too would their work evolve, becoming similar to his.

The first statement hasn't yet come to fruition. Although there are several offshoots of the Method, the way graduates work looks very similar to what Dr Feldenkrais was doing with his students. The second statement is certainly true in that there are indeed many more practitioners who are discovering the importance of internal experience and awareness in learning or skill acquisition.

When Dr Feldenkrais started the San Francisco Professional Training Program in 1975, he expected his students to take his teaching into their own professions, transforming the way they taught, counseled and performed, rather than copy his work directly.

He said, 'You can't teach anybody anything, you can only create conditions in which they can learn.'

Having recently returned to teaching music more traditionally after many years of working as a Feldenkrais practitioner and Assistant Trainer, I see a great need for bringing Dr Feldenkrais' brilliant ideas on learning into our schools, playing fields and all areas of education. Much of the educating of students is done by instructing them rather than providing guidance for discovery. In this manner, teachers 'teach' rather than create conditions for learning.

My study and practice of the Feldenkrais Method enables me to teach music very differently than how I was taught. My hope is that helping teachers and institutions to create better learning conditions which are based on self-inquiry, maturation and growth could be a very worthy contribution to humanity."

I asked my friend and colleague Candy Conino, a Feldenkrais Assistant Trainer, whether she thought the method would survive, and she said:

"The Feldenkrais Method will carry on into the future because it can handle any and all challenges.

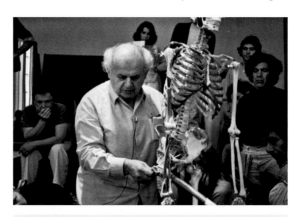

Figure 24.2
Moshe Feldenkrais teaching, San Francisco.

As a practitioner I have thrown every challenge I can discover or invent at this work. It does not disappoint or fall short. This Method is strong, resilient, flexible, forgiving and somehow made even more powerful by creative initiatives. It flourishes on a diet of basic human attributes and desires: observation; connection; adaptation; articulation; collaboration; and respect. If we embrace the principles of the Feldenkrais Method and integrate them fully into our lives, we will all have a clarity of intention and the flexible minds necessary to negotiate the unknown, and benefit from the opportunities of the future."

Chandler Stevens, a young student in Dr Jeff Haller's Feldenkrais Training Academy in Seattle, shared this:

"The Method itself seems to be in a precarious situation. It's big and challenging and vast, applicable in some way to every human on earth. And yet it requires a rare level of willingness to explore, an appreciation of nuance, and a patience with the not-yet-known.

I think of a line from Gregory Bateson's introduction to his book, *Mind and Nature* (2002), 'There seems to be something like a Gresham's law of cultural evolution according to which the oversimplified ideas will always displace the sophisticated and the vulgar and hateful will always displace the beautiful. And yet the beautiful persists.'

The Method is beautiful. As practitioners we have an incredible responsibility to become better stewards of it, to do the hard work of bringing it to a world in desperate need of the qualities it cultivates in each of us."

Anastasi Siotas, an experienced practitioner and soon-to-be minted Feldenkrais Trainer who grew up in Australia and practices in many locations, offers another perspective:

"For over 50 years the Feldenkrais Method has continuously evolved into new fields of application.

First, second and third-generation Trainers have faithfully transmitted and developed the rich legacy of materials that Dr Moshe Feldenkrais presciently left behind. His audio and video recordings, along with his seminal books and writings, are a rich treasure. The inspiration for developing the group lesson format *Awareness through Movement* came from Moshe's desire to spread his discoveries to as many people as possible. He achieved a modicum of success in his Swiss and Israeli weekly radio broadcasts. Today, however, using the Internet, teachers are able to reach countless numbers across the globe, creating ever broader ripples of exposure to his work.

I recently taught in the first teacher training program in China and will soon teach in the first Russian training program. I feel optimistic about our future because of this growing global interest and am secure in the knowledge of how effectively Feldenkrais lessons can rebuild neural connections. Instead of being pushed toward the precipice of flight/fright sympathetic dominance, low vagal tone, and low heart rate variability, each Feldenkrais experience offers a panacea of mindful action. Whether imagining or doing, we monitor and self-adjust the often-invisible expenditure of energy to its most conservative and therefore restorative level. The Feldenkrais Method has offered me concrete experiences that have led to better decision making for improved self-care for myself, my loved ones, and my students. Now, more than ever, we need ways of moving, sensing, feeling, and thinking that create harmony and promote the circuitry of deeper connection with ourselves, other living beings, and our planet."

Chris Murray, a long-time student and irrepressible Feldenkrais aficionado proposed:

"Has the world been too comfortable to fully appreciate the Feldenkrais Method? It sprang from strife, war and injury, from a refugee who had to deal with

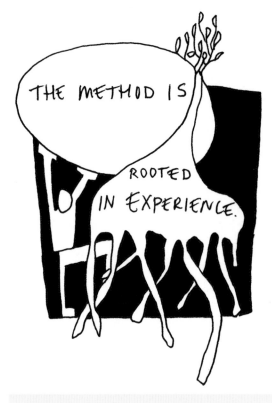

Figure 24.3
The Method is rooted in experience.

Courtesy of Tiffany Sankary 2014. *Feldenkrais Illustrated: The Art of Learning,* Movement and Creativity Press

systemic racism and prejudice; it was built for judo, for combat, for the most challenging conceivable environments. The growing difficulties and anxieties we are facing today will cause the genius of this Method to shine even brighter.

Distance learning is here to stay. There has been system-wide change as Feldenkrais teachers have overhauled their practices for the online environment. Maybe this involves some new friction, but less than expected – and I love inviting friends to class from all over the planet (one morning recently

we had Hong Kong, Italy, Germany, Switzerland and South Africa all represented).

How can we get the medical profession more deeply engaged with the Feldenkrais Method? Let us, together with neurologists and other doctors, psychiatrists, and performance experts, unpack its unique insights into brain function. Maybe someday, with fMRI studies or other studies more suited to register the benefits of Feldenkrais. Might we even find philanthropy to help us make Feldenkrais accessible for everyone in a sustainable way? It's time to invest in wellness for all communities, not just those who can afford it."

I had the fortuitous opportunity to interview Mia Segal, Moshe Feldenkrais' first assistant, a judo black belt, and veteran teacher in what he originally called "Human Body Sculpting." Her testimony made me think how it is often by looking back that we can better determine our future. She recalls:

"I had been an Alexander teacher, and Moshe suggested I join him in his work, so I went to watch him give someone a lesson and it had a big impact on me. I can still describe the room and its details to this day, and I said to him, 'I would like to join you, but first I want to come and learn from you.' Thus began many years of learning, working and a special friendship that touched and enriched me and my family.

His stories about Judo and Eastern philosophy inspired us and this was one of the reasons why, after ten years, I took a break and went with my family to Japan. During this three-year period of time we learned judo, Japanese and made wonderful friends. Before we left, Moshe came to visit us, realizing one of his dreams when we introduced him to great Japanese judo masters. Returning to Israel, I resumed my work with Moshe.

In 1975 Thomas Hanna, founder of the Human Psychology Society, invited us to present Moshe's

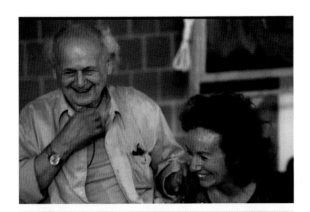

Figure 24.4
Moshe Feldenkrais and Mia Segal in San Francisco.

method in San Francisco. We discussed at length what name to give to the work that would describe what we were doing. The expression Moshe used for the process was shichlul hayecholet, which in Hebrew means 'refinement of abilities.'

Later, when I heard President Barack Obama inspire a whole nation with the words, 'Yes, we can!' I said to myself, this describes exactly what we do.

There is no need to add to Moshe's Method as he presented it in San Francisco. It is the complete Method, the essence is there, in theory and practice. However, we can go on refining it to higher levels. The Method is ready, the world is ready, and there are many good teachers.

I believe that this Method should be taught to all, beginning in childhood, just like the ABCs. Children will grow up aware that they are in charge of their movements and that these are metaphors for their greater abilities. They will grow up knowing how to take responsibility, make choices, and have the power and joy that comes with the practice of using their 'Yes I can!'"

And finally, this from Larry Goldfarb, a seasoned Feldenkrais Trainer, who studied with Feldenkrais in the Amherst Professional Training Program in the early 1980s:

"My dream is that there will be Feldenkrais teachers in neighborhoods around the world. Just like you know when to call upon the local piano teacher or plumber, you'll know to contact your nearby Feldenkrais teacher when you want to improve your coordination, to recover or improve your ability to do things you love – be that cooking, crocheting or canoeing, walking, running or jumping, playing a sport or a musical instrument, or playing with your children or grandchildren."

I hope that this book has convinced you that the Feldenkrais Method, with all of its vast applications, evolutions and iterations, is not only thriving throughout the world, but will continue to remain an essential and vital component of the lives of future generations.

References

Bateson, G. 2002. *Mind and Nature*. Hampton Press, London.

Working the Extensors of the Back *Awareness Through Movement* Audio Lesson taught by Anastasi Siotas

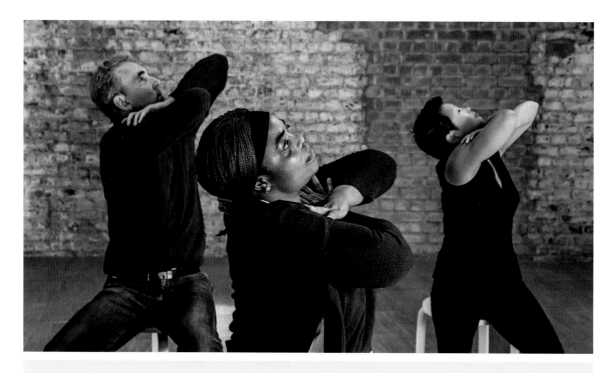

Figure 24.5
"There are no limits to our possibilities." Moshe Feldenkrais.

Feldenkrais Access: Article Archive

Curated by David Zemach-Bersin, this growing archive houses over 250 Feldenkrais-related articles. Topics include Dr Moshe Feldenkrais, chronic pain, back pain, research, general health, the performing arts, and more. Over 20 articles have been translated into Spanish.

There is a direct link to the Archives; you need to submit your email to access it, but you are not required to sign up for the email list unless you wish to do so.

www.feldenkraisaccess.com/offers/or4tCxy2/checkout

Selected Reading

Alon, R. 2018. *Mindful Spontaneity: Lessons in the Feldenkrais Method*. North Atlantic Books, Berkeley, CA.

Doidge, N. 2015. *The Brain's Way of Healing: Remarkable Discoveries and Recoveries from the Frontiers of Neuroplasticity*. Viking Books, New York.

Doidge, N. 2007. *The Brain that Changes Itself: Stories of Personal Triumph from the Frontiers of Brain Science*. Penguin, New York.

Feldenkrais, M. 2010. In: E. Beringer (ed.) *Embodied Wisdom: The Collected Papers of Moshe Feldenkrais*. North Atlantic Books, Berkeley, CA.

Feldenkrais, M. 1972. *Awareness Through Movement: Health Exercises for Personal Growth*. Harper & Row, New York.

Feldenkrais, M. 1993. *Body Awareness as Healing Therapy: The Case of Nora,* 2nd edn. North Atlantic Books, Berkeley, CA.

Feldenkrais, M. 1998. *The Potent Self: A Study of Spontaneity and Compulsion,* Reprint. Frog Limited & Somatic Resources, Berkeley, CA.

Feldenkrais, M., Soloway, T., Baniel, A., Krauss, J. (eds.). 2013. *Alexander Yanai Lessons*. International Feldenkrais Federation, Paris.

Feldenkrais, M. 2002. *Body and Mature Behavior: A Study of Gravitation, Anxiety, Sex and Learning*. Frog Ltd/Somatic Resources, Berkeley, CA.

Feldenkrais, M. 2019. *The Elusive Obvious*, Reprint. North Atlantic Books/Somatic Resources, San Francisco, CA.

Reese, M. 2015. *Moshe Feldenkrais: A Life in Movement*. ReeseKress Somatics Press, San Rafael, CA.

Rywerant, Y. 2000. *Acquiring the Feldenkrais Profession*. El-Or, Tel Aviv.

Wildman, F. 2016. *The Busy Person's Guide to Easier Movement*. CreateSpace Independent Publishing.

Zemach-Bersin, D. 1990. *Relaxercise: The Easy New Way to Health and Fitness*. HarperOne, New York

Research about the Feldenkrais Method

IFF Academy *Feldenkrais Research Journal* https://feldenkrais-method.org/research/
IFF Research Bibliography https://feldenkrais-method.org/en/research/reference-database/
The Australian Feldenkrais Guild Research webpage https://www.feldenkrais.org.au/research

The Feldenkrais® Educational Foundation of North America (FEFNA)
FEFNA supports theoretically grounded research that extends and advances the *Feldenkrais Method*.
https://feldenkrais.com/feldenkrais-educational-foundation-north-america/

Locate a Feldenkrais Practitioner Worldwide

The Feldenkrais Guild UK http://www.feldenkrais.co.uk/
The Feldenkrais Guild of North America https://feldenkrais.com/
The Australian Feldenkrais Guild https://www.feldenkrais.org.au
https://feldenkrais-method.org/iff/member-organizations/

PERMISSIONS

The editors gratefully acknowledge the International Feldenkrais® Federation's permission to use the following photos and audio files in the book. They appreciate the IFF Archive of the Feldenkrais Method's mandate to preserve the legacy of Dr Moshe Feldenkrais by making so many materials available to practitioners as well as to the public. https://feldenkrais-method.org

The editors gratefully acknowledge the following for the valuable contribution of their photos and illustrations.

The Israel Museum, Jerusalem
Figure 1.2

Tiffany Sankary, *Movement and Creativity*
Figures 9.1, 13.1, 13.2, 22.1, 22.2, 22.3, 22.4, 24.1, 24.2

Moshe Feldenkrais
Figure 7.5

Dave Susko @Foto Phreak
Figure 17.3

Human Kinetics
Figures 18:2, 18.3, 18.4, 18.5

Josh Riemer, Unsplash
Figure 3.2

Chapter 1: Who Was Moshe Feldenkrais?
"Moshe Feldenkrais in the 1930s"

Chapter 4: Training Feldenkrais® Teachers
"Moshe Feldenkrais teaching Functional Integration in Amherst 1981"
Photography by Jerry Karzen

Chapter 6: The Feldenkrais Method®, Science, and Spirituality: A Historical Perspective
"Moshe Feldenkrais teaching in Freiburg"
Photography by Michael Wolgensinger
"Judo Throw: Moshe Feldenkrais with Mikonosuke Kawaishi, who together founded the Jiu-Jitsu Club of France, 1938"

Chapter 7: Moshe Dō: From Martial Art to Feldenkrais® Art

"Instinctive defense against a knife stab by Moshe Feldenkrais, 1930"

© International Feldenkrais® Federation, Paris, France. All rights reserved.

"Knife technique (Moshe Feldenkrais on the *left*)"

© International Feldenkrais® Federation, Paris, France. All rights reserved.

"Hadaka Jime (Naked Hands choke; Moshe Feldenkrais on the *right*)"

© International Feldenkrais® Federation, Paris, France. All rights reserved.

"Moshe Feldenkrais and Kawaishi 'breaking" knees'

© International Feldenkrais® Federation, Paris, France. All rights reserved.

Chapter 19: Somatic Education: Feldenkrais® and Pilates

"Moshe Feldenkrais using rollers to work with a child"

© International Feldenkrais® Federation, Paris, France. All rights reserved.

Photography by Michael Wolgensinger

Chapter 24: A Future Vision of the Feldenkrais Method®

"Moshe Feldenkrais Teaching with Skeleton, San Francisco"

© International Feldenkrais® Federation, Paris, France. All rights reserved.

Photography by © Bob Knighton

"Moshe Feldenkrais and Mia Segal portrait Amherst"

© International Feldenkrais® Federation, Paris, France. All rights reserved.

Photography by © Bob Knighton

Contemporary Image

© International Feldenkrais® Federation and Robert Golden. All rights reserved.

Inside cover

Contemporary Image

© International Feldenkrais® Federation and Robert Golden. All rights reserved.

https://feldenkrais-method.org/

INDEX

Note: Page numbers followed by f indicate figure